Her Body, Her Baby

Real Stories of Autonomy in Childbirth

By

Dr. Michael J. Hervey II MD

This book is for anyone who believes birth should be better—for patients, providers, families, and the system itself. It speaks truth, invites reflection, and dares to imagine a future where birth is safe, human, and healing.

For Patients

- **The first-time parent**, excited but unprepared, stepping into the unknown of labor and delivery.
- **The survivor**, carrying trauma, grief, or disappointment from past birth experiences—and ready to reclaim their story.
- **The family member or partner**, seeking a way to open up honest conversations about birth, expectations, and emotional needs.
- **The advocate**, searching for tools to make informed, autonomous decisions in an often-disempowering system.

For Providers

- **The student or early-career clinician**, eager to find meaning, impact, and purpose in a broken system.
- **The seasoned provider**, burnt out and disillusioned, who once believed they could make a difference—and still wants to.

- **The "old guard" physician**, struggling to adapt to a new era of shared decision-making, informed consent, and empowered patients.
- **The nurse**, who stands by patients in their most vulnerable moments, offering comfort, courage, and care.
- **The midwife**, often undervalued, yet central to safe, personalized, and powerful birth experiences.

For the System Itself

- **Healthcare leaders**, tasked with redesigning maternal care to meet both the ancient wisdom and modern needs of childbirth.
- **Policy makers and institutions**, wrestling with how to support collaborative care: OBs, MFMs, midwives, hospitalists, and doulas—*together*.
- **Hospital systems**, navigating outdated protocols and a rising call for home births, VBACs, breech deliveries, and true patient autonomy.

For the World Beyond the Delivery Room

- **For the unborn**, whose lives deserve thoughtful, ethical, and compassionate care.
- **For the curious**, even those far removed from birth but close to someone who isn't—this is for you too.

This Book Is for Change

It doesn't end with the last page—it begins. Let this be the start of hard conversations, system shifts, healing journeys, and radical reimagining of what birth can and should be.

Buy it. Read it. Share it. Let's start the change—together.

Contents

Dedication

To the women who have given my life its greatest meaning —
This book is born from your love.

To Ellie Tan, CNM — my wife, my partner, the finest Midwife I have ever known.
Your hands heal, your heart leads, and your wisdom lifts every life you touch.
It is your quiet strength that shows me, daily, how to serve with grace.

To my daughter and dearest friend, Kieara Hervey —
You are the light that pushes me to be better, love harder, and believe more deeply.
Your pure heart and fearless spirit remind me what true possibility looks like.

To my mother and my sister —
Your unwavering love has been my shelter, my compass, my courage.
Without your belief in me, I would not be standing here, living this calling.

And to the Premier Team, both past and present —
Thank you for your hands, hearts, and endless devotion to a

dream greater than any of us.

This work carries your spirit, every single day.

This book is for all of you —

The ones who taught me that honoring a woman's voice, her strength, her story —

It is the most sacred work I will ever do.

Preface

Lunch had ended, and I grabbed my computer from my desk to open the next chart: a new patient, 28 weeks pregnant, first-time mother (G1P0). The details intrigued me. At this stage in pregnancy, had she been receiving care elsewhere, or was this a transfer due to some significant delay? I wondered what surprises awaited behind the next door.

Her chart revealed two blood pressure readings: 180/100 and a repeat of 160/90. My curiosity deepened as I prepared to meet her.

Her name is Salima. Age: 30. First pregnancy.
I knocked on the exam room door.
"Come in," a raspy voice called out.

Inside, I found a petite Caucasian woman, about five feet tall, 110 lbs, and visibly pregnant with a modest bump. She wore a light summer dress with a V-neck that revealed a surgical scar running down her mid-sternum. Sitting elevated on the exam table, she radiated confidence. Her husband stood nearby—a towering, muscular man with dark olive skin. Despite his imposing presence, his shy demeanor softened the room's atmosphere. It was clear, though, that Salima was the commanding presence in the relationship.

I introduced myself formally. *"I'm Dr. Hervey. Welcome! How did you hear about us?"* I always ask this of new patients, and Im curious how they find us since we've never advertised. *"My aunt recommended you,"* she replied. *"She's a Midwife in Northern Phoenix."* I pressed further. *"Who's your aunt?"*

When she named her, I immediately recognized the name. Her aunt was a renowned Midwife, an elder revered in the community who could command a standing ovation in a clinical setting. I was humbled.

I transitioned into my customary introduction. *"Let me explain my approach to care,"* I began. *"What I value most is providing good care and a good experience. That means I won't dictate what to do or how to do it. My role is to educate and offer options. I will not walk into your environment and tell you what I am going to do to you. Anyone doing something to you without your consent—that would be assault, and I will never do that."*

"For instance, I won't walk in and say, 'I'm going to check your cervix now.' Instead, I'll offer you an exam. You may ask, 'Am I okay? Is the baby, okay?' If both answers are affirmative, you have the right and responsibility to decline the exam if you choose. It's your body, your choice, as long as you are safe."

As I spoke, Salima began to cry. Her tears caught me off guard. She was a first-time mother—what had I said to elicit such a strong reaction? I handed her a tissue and paused. *"What's wrong? Did I say something upsetting?"* I asked gently.

She sighed deeply. *"No, everything you said was perfect. I see why my aunt wanted me to come to you. You're a breath of fresh air."*

Out of the corner of my eye, I noticed her husband smiling, his eyes glistening. I thanked her for her kind words but pressed on. *"I'm curious. Why are you starting care so late in the third trimester?"*

Her composure broke, and the sobs came. Through tears, she shared her story.

"I was born with a severe coarctation of the aorta, requiring four major surgeries throughout my life. Most of my descending aorta is now a Gore-Tex graft. These surgeries caused ischemic injury, leaving me with chronic kidney disease—Stage III or IV. My blood pressure is extremely high, and due to the graft, the readings may not even be accurate."

Salima continued, *"For two trimesters, I've searched for a provider willing to care for me. Six different doctors turned me away, saying I was too high-risk. Even two MFM specialists questioned why I got pregnant, berated my cardiologist for clearing me, and told me I could die. Every day, I wake up terrified—unsure if my baby or I will survive this pregnancy. I feel judged for wanting to be a mother, for dreaming of a vaginal birth. I'm scared and alone."*

Her story was heart-wrenching. I allowed her and her husband time to console each other while I gathered my thoughts. Once ready, I completed her history and physical, and began crafting a plan.

"Salima," I said gently, *"I recommend admitting you to the hospital immediately. We'll have an MFM consult tomorrow, gather your cardiac records, and develop a plan to keep both you and your baby safe. I can't promise how this will end, but I'll give you, my best. I'll advocate for you and respect your wishes where possible. That said, we must prepare for preeclampsia, premature delivery, or even a cesarean."*

Her tears returned, but this time, they seemed mixed with relief. She and her husband hugged me before heading to the hospital for admission. I called MFM, cardiology, charge nurses, and residents to ensure everyone understood her complex case. Salima didn't just need a doctor—she needed an ally. And that's where true patient care begins.

Salima's story highlights the challenges and biases in modern pregnancy care, where patients with unique needs or unconventional choices often face judgment and systemic barriers. When Salima sought help, she didn't need avoidance or criticism—she needed empathy, advocacy, and action. Instead of rallying around her to provide the care she deserved, the healthcare community hesitated, paralyzed by fears of liability and unfamiliarity with her situation.

This delay left her vulnerable, navigating a system that should have supported her but alienated her and her family. Salima's experience is a stark reminder that genuine patient-centered care means being a *"soft landing"* where patients feel safe, supported, and respected. It's about recognizing their autonomy and choices while ensuring their safety, even when those choices challenge the norms of traditional practice. Her story urges providers to move beyond fear and judgment, prioritizing compassion and advocacy for every patient.

A critical issue in modern healthcare, particularly in pregnancy care, is that biases, systemic barriers, and risk-averse practices often overshadow the patient-centered approach that should be the foundation of medicine:

1. Empathy and Advocacy: Salima's experience underscores the need for healthcare providers to prioritize empathy over judgment. Advocacy for the patient's needs, irrespective of how *"different"* their situation or choices might appear, is a fundamental aspect of ethical care.

2. Breaking Barriers: The structural and interpersonal barriers that prevent patients from accessing timely and appropriate care

are a significant concern. Providers must actively work to minimize these barriers, whether from institutional policies, biases, or fear of liability.

3. Safety and Autonomy: Acknowledging and respecting a patient's autonomy—while ensuring their safety—is a delicate but essential balance. The focus should remain on enabling informed choices rather than imposing a specific course of action.

4. Reexamining Provider Roles: The imagery of healthcare providers "standing boldly and loudly in front of patients" suggests a performative aspect of care that can sometimes alienate rather than support. It calls for introspection and a shift toward being a "soft landing"—a trusted partner who provides care with humility, understanding, and respect for the patient's experience.

Let's look at the healthcare education system and how it contributed to Salima's Story.

Chapter 1

Shifting Landscapes: Medical Education, Obstetrical Practice, and Economic Pressures

---

The landscape of medical education, Obstetrical practice, and physician compensation has undergone profound transformations over the last few decades. These shifts have deeply impacted my career and personal experience in healthcare, especially in Obstetric.

Reflecting on the trends in medical education for graduates, the evolution of Obstetrical training and practice, and the economic pressures of inflation, I find these interconnected challenges shaping my approach to modern medicine.

My Observations on Trends in Medical Education

The number of students pursuing medicine appears to have declined. Many are drawn to corporate, entertainment, financial, technology, and social media industries that offer comparable or better financial outcomes with potentially less grueling work. These fields provide more immediate access to wealth and status than the demanding and prolonged medical training journey. Yet, despite these challenges, medical education continues to evolve, driven by the ongoing need for healthcare professionals and the enduring appeal of a career that combines science and service.

As our graduates' shift from innovative medical roles, many others prefer to maintain the status quo. They avoid drawing attention to themselves or their field and focus on being recognized for strong clinical and ethical work. Innovators who bring fresh ideas are often those less intimidated by the system's hierarchy.

My Experiences in Obstetrical Practice and Education

Obstetrics represents a unique blend of real medicine and personalized care. During my training in Family Medicine, I gained invaluable exposure to general medicine and continuity care clinics. This exposure allowed me to stand in and fill the void that less personalized care offers. Thus, patients often came to me because they needed someone to trust and share their problems with. However, in emergencies, trust shifted to a universal reliance on competence. In an acute heart attack, for example, patients focused solely on survival, placing their faith in the closest available provider, regardless of background.

When I transitioned to Obstetric, filling the gap and providing personalized care was easy. I became a soft landing for many looking to enter the healthcare system. At the same time, those individuals were also looking for competency in clinical knowledge and skills. I experienced firsthand the high-stakes and high-intensity nature of the field. My training included rapid decision-making, emergency surgeries, and managing life-threatening scenarios such as hemorrhages requiring massive transfusions and ICU admissions. These experiences have shaped my practice and understanding of today's Obstetrical training.

After four years of high-risk and highly complex medical care, many Obstetrical providers transition to practice that avoids high-risk cases. They now limit their practices to low-risk patients, a trend contributing to a decline in the day-to-day acuity addressed during training. For example, vaginal breech birth is losing footing in the medical community, as well as forceps-assisted deliveries, accretas, amongst many others.

For example, board certified OB/GYN hospitalist was called upon to assist with an acute focal accreta. The accreta was undiagnosed, the baby was born and mom was bleeding; two liters of blood was lost. The surgeon caught by surprise called out to the hospitalist to assist for the safety and well being of the mom. The Hospitalist declined his/her assistance and rather sent a Physician Assistant to retract for the surgeon. In the end over four liters of blood was senselessly lost adding to the morbidity of the patients care.

Reflections on Limited Specialization in Obstetrics

The generalist approach to OB-GYN training often leaves physicians less prepared for complex cases. In my training, I performed forceps-assisted deliveries only a few times, gaining most of my proficiency during Family Medicine training and through subsequent practice under senior supervision. Similarly, I encountered only a handful of breech deliveries despite their appropriateness in certain settings. Many teachings faculty simply recommended cesarean sections for these cases, and some even preferred all twin deliveries to be performed surgically.

This evolution in practice has led to sub specialization within Obstetrics. High-risk Obstetrics is increasingly handled by Maternal-Fetal Medicine (MFM) specialists, who now face decisions about whether to focus on clinical or surgical roles. These trends highlight a growing stratification within the field, where generalists focus on low-acuity cases. At the same time, subspecialists manage complex scenarios such as placenta accreta or pregnancies in patients with extreme BMIs or multiple prior cesarean sections.

To give a real-life example of this dire nature of this risk-based shift where providers electively avoid standard care; I was told of a patient who was scheduled by MFM to be delivered due to maternal obesity. The goal was 38 wk. delivery via c-section. The hospitalist that happened to be on call the day of surgery refused the case- "I don't feel comfortable operating/ delivering a patient this size". The case was canceled, and rescheduled for another day. Once again, the surgery was met with the same response by another hospitalist; the case was rescheduled. Once more the case was scheduled and confirmed with the hospital 10 days later than the initial date. The patient presented complaining of decreased fetal movement, but I am here for my scheduled surgery. Upon attempt to find heart beat- there was none. The baby had passed away. A loss that could have been avoid had the hospitalist worked to the fullest of his/her scope – what he/she was trained.

My Perspective on the Role of Midwifery

Midwifery care has seen a powerful and inspiring resurgence over the past several decades. Since 1990, the number of practicing Midwives has grown dramatically, and the impact on maternity care is undeniable. In the United States alone, the proportion of births attended by Midwives increased from approximately 3.9% in 1990 to 12% in 2021—a more than threefold rise that speaks volumes about the trust and demand placed in this model of care.

Midwifery represents a deeply human, patient-centered approach to childbirth. It has become a vital alternative to traditional Obstetric care, especially for individuals with low-risk pregnancies. Certified Nurse-M Midwives (CNMs) and other Midwifery professionals provide exceptional care grounded in relationship, respect, and a personalized experience that prioritizes both the parent and babys physical, emotional, and psychological well -being. This model fills critical gaps in our healthcare system and reflects a shift toward empowering patients to make informed, values-aligned choices about their care.

Significantly, Midwives are also expanding their scope. I have seen Midwives take on the care of some higher-risk patients- this is done well with collaborative care model, including those pursuing vaginal births after cesarean (TOLACs).

While low-risk scenarios highlight the growing confidence and competency within Midwifery, many Midwives collaborate with physicians and hospitals to ensure that risk is responsibly managed, always with the patient's wishes and safety at the center.

The surge in Midwifery is not just a response to medical necessity—it's also driven by real opportunity. Families are increasingly willing to invest in birth experiences that are personalized, empowering, and centered around continuity of care. Patients may pay between $7,000 and $10,000 for Midwifery-led care that prioritizes them as individuals, rather than as numbers in a high-volume hospital system. This model offers low-volume, high-touch care, and many Midwives can operate with financial sustainability, some even outside the constraints of traditional insurance systems, while maintaining intense patient satisfaction.

In a healthcare system that often favors intervention over intuition, Midwifery offers a grounded, human-centered alternative. Midwives are reclaiming their rightful place in maternity care—and transforming it for the better.

Yet with this resurgence comes a caution: when Midwifery practice drifts toward overconfidence, poor collaboration, and unchecked extremes of patient autonomy, it can lead to serious harm. Balance is not optional—it is essential.

Inflation and Physician Salaries: My Perspective

Economic pressures further complicate the practice of medicine. While nominally high, physician salaries have struggled to keep pace with inflation, especially when adjusted to rising practice costs. As an Obstetrician, I face unique financial challenges, including the high cost of malpractice insurance due to the inherent risks of childbirth. Physician income growth has been relatively stagnant compared to other well-compensated industries like technology, finance, and law, where salaries have outpaced inflation. Many physicians will invest in passive income streams to offset the losses incurred as dedicated providers. Arizona has consistently lagged behind the country in compensation for child birth. In comparison to the self-pay concierge opportunities of birth centers and the home birth Midwives ($7000-10000). Physician compensation for a vaginal birth ranges $800- $2500. This payment is a global payment for nine months of maternity care and varies very little. For a cesarean add $500 to $1000 more at best.

Industries like technology benefit from market-driven salaries, performance-based incentives, and flexible work environments. In contrast, I—and many of my colleagues—operate within rigid reimbursement systems and face increasing administrative burdens. More regulations with lower compensation for the total time and effort given. The stability of a medical career is offset by economic pressures that constrain real earnings and influence career choices, particularly in high-risk specialties like Obstetrics.

CONCLUSION

The intertwined challenges of medical education, Obstetrical practice, and economic realities underscore the complexities of modern medicine. These challenges drive a wedge into a practitioner's will and desire to allow autonomy in practice to flourish. While medical education continues to attract both American and foreign graduates, the evolving nature of Obstetrical training and practice reflects a growing divide between generalists and subspecialists. This divide opens up the opportunity for Midwifery and personalized care to take root. This is a positive aspect of Obstetrics, but it leads to a greater divide in the culture of birth work and financial unrest. The economic pressures of inflation and stagnant physician salaries further complicate these dynamics. By focusing on trust-based patient relationships and maintaining full-scope practices, I strive to navigate these challenges while delivering high-quality care that meets the diverse needs of my patients. Autonomy is rewarding but costly in time.

Chapter 2

Their Body, Their Choice: A Lesson in Compassionate Care

Habid's Choice

Morning rounds had just finished, and we had gathered as a team to review the board, sign out the night cases, and assign new providers to each patient. At Maricopa County Hospital, *"The COPA"* sign-out was a ritual where the attending physicians would gather with the team and drill the resident running the board, typically an upper-level resident. The exercise, a high-pressure quiz-and-response session, was designed to prepare us for the oral board examinations and was a rite of passage every resident experienced multiple times during training.

As the morning rounds wound down, a call came in from triage: an active laboring patient had arrived, and a resident assignment was needed. The patient's name was Habid.

Typically, when this occurred, there was a systematic process to determine who would manage the patient. A provider without another laboring patient would be first in line. If the patient is at low risk, a first-year or a rotating provider (Family Medicine or Emergency Medicine) would be tasked to manage the patient. In this instance, the room fell silent. Audible gasps and palpable tension filled the air. I was a second-year resident, experienced enough to manage most situations but still too naive to grasp the weight of the name *"Habid."* Confusion clouded my mind as I watched seasoned doctors and even the program director exchange uneasy glances. On some faces, a disdain for the name Habid arose, and others were angry and afraid. Finally, the silence broke:

"I will not take care of that patient," declared the program director, her voice firm with finality.

A pregnant chief resident quickly echoed, *"I cannot be involved in her care either. I mentally cannot handle that kind of stress."*

Many others followed suit, one after another. Nearly the entire room refused to care for this patient. I was amazed and in shock; awe had overtaken me by the willingness to neglect care. What on earth could be so devastating that no one was willing to assist this refugee woman in need? Was it her race, nationality, or other?

Still unsure of the full context but recognizing the urgency, I stepped forward, filling the void left by the refusal of others. *"I'll take care of her,"* I said, my voice steady, though uncertainty swirled within me. *"Great,"* echoed the team, but an attending provider was still needed to chaperone my sophomoric skill set.

Dr. Jules was called in from the clinics. She was the only attending physician in the hospital or clinic willing to assist with Habid's care. Another provider electively chose to see Dr. Jules' clinic patients instead. It was at this point, sitting with Dr. Jules, that I learned the back story and why anxiety was so high around Habid and her care for this pregnancy.

Approximately 13 months earlier, Habid, a gravida-5 para-4 Somali woman, had been admitted to the labor unit. She was a refugee with limited English proficiency and had been in the U.S. for less than a year. Habid was truly a stranger in a strange land, and having delivered four children vaginally in Somalia, her labor was expected to progress smoothly.

But her labor didn't go as planned. It was anything but smooth.

Well into the labor, Habid's fetal heart tracing began showing signs of fetal distress, and there were concerning decelerations. The reactivity and the fetal well-being began to decline. Despite all resuscitative measures, contractions were ineffective in making an adequate change. Thus, her cervix remained unchanged. With every bit of reason, Habid was offered a cesarean section, but she outright refused. The situation became dire: meconium began draining, the fetal heart tracing flattened, and the baby showed no signs of improvement.

The team contacted everyone for guidance, calling on a broad support network. This was an unusual and complex situation that few had likely encountered before. Yet, they remained focused, seeking input from medical professionals and community members with more U.S. experience, including the hospital chaplain and even the ethics committee. Together, they pleaded with her to consent to an emergency C-section. Still, she refused.

In the end, her baby died. She labored and delivered a stillborn baby girl. The grief in the room was overwhelming—hers, ours, everyone's.

Now, here she was, a year later, pregnant with her sixth pregnancy, soon-to-be fifth child. The memories of that tragic event resonated so profoundly that even the mention of her name sent shockwaves through the team. The refusal to care for her was not just a refusal to relive that trauma—it was a judgment on her choices, perceived as *"evil"* by those who couldn't comprehend her decisions.

But regardless of her past, she was here now, a laboring patient in need. Dr. Jules and I stood in the gap and committed to her care. We were determined to provide a soft landing for Habid concerning her current and past decisions. It's her body, it's her baby!

Under Dr. Jule's guidance, we delivered her baby vaginally. The experience was profoundly humbling. Through tears, Habid expressed heartfelt gratitude.

The cultural context surrounding her decisions began to come into focus for me. In Somalia, cesarean sections are often perceived as a death sentence. These surgeries are performed with the patient wrapped in a burial shroud, and families prepare for the high possibility of death. Sanitation and sterility are at an all-time low in Habid's homeland, and there is no blood for transfusions readily available. For Habid, choosing not to risk a C-section wasn't about defiance or recklessness—it was about survival. She had a family to protect, a husband, and four children depending on her in a foreign country without an extended family. Her decision to refuse surgery during her fifth pregnancy wasn't negligent; it was the most informed choice she could make within the framework of her cultural beliefs and experiences.

This epiphany reshaped my perspective on patient care early in Obstetrics. My role wasn't to judge a patient's decisions or impose my values on them, but to offer help and provide care with empathy and respect, no matter the circumstances.

Boundless Duty

I encountered a similar lesson while working in an ER on a reservation. Two brothers, intoxicated and enraged, had fought over a woman. The elder brother had bludgeoned the younger one unconscious with a 4x4. Both ended up in the same ER, the severely injured brother needing urgent stabilization and helicopter transport to a trauma center. At the same time, the aggressor was restrained and shouting threats from a nearby stretcher.

Tasked with suturing the aggressor's minor wounds, I felt a wave of anger. Yet, I forced myself to do my best work, suppress my disgust, and provide him with needed care. It was a defining moment, teaching me that my emotions and judgments had no place in the care I provided.

Conclusion

Refugee care and care-on-reservations are unique experiences in American medicine. These populations' cultural beliefs, traditional practices, and systemic disparities often challenge conventional healthcare norms. Yet, they also highlight the importance of understanding and respecting a patient's perspective.

In Somali culture, female circumcision remains a practice despite its illegality in the U.S. In the Hmong community, a shaman's approval is sometimes required before life-saving interventions can proceed. These situations test our systems and ethics and illuminate the essence of patient-centered care.

The greatest epiphany from these experiences has been the recognition that every patient deserves autonomy. Their body, their beliefs, their choices. My role is not to judge but to provide the best care possible, to be a soft-landing spot where they feel safe, understood, and respected.

For Salima, Habid, the brothers in the ER, and every patient I've cared for—it's their body, their choice, their life.

Chapter 3

Empowered Birth: Balancing Patient Autonomy and Medical Safety

In my practice, I meet a patient like Salima, who breaks down in tears nearly every week. My introduction resonates with the mother, grandmother, sisters, extended family, and even the baby's father. These moments are both poignant and transformative.

Allow me to introduce my clinic philosophy and care model:

What I care about most is good care and a good experience. This means I am not the provider who walks into any environment and dictates what must be done. Instead, I am the provider who walks into your space to provide options, empowering you to decide what is best for your body, your baby, and your family, as long as you are safe.

"I tell every patient: anything done to you without your consent is assault. My job is not to assault you. My job is to educate you because educated people make educated decisions. You are the boss as long as you and your baby are safe."

To illustrate, I would never walk into your labor environment and say, *"I'm going to check your cervix,"* without understanding where you are mentally, emotionally, physically, spiritually, culturally, religiously, or socially. Instead, you should ask me, *"Am I okay?"* If my reply is yes, your next question might be, *"Is my baby, okay?"* If both are affirmative, you have the right and responsibility to communicate your preferences, such as declining an exam. Your words should be respected by me and by every provider you encounter.

Similarly, I would not dictate interventions like breaking your water or starting Pitocin. Instead, I would offer options. I might say, *"You've been at six centimeters for over six hours without change. Option one is to do nothing—move around, use a birthing ball, get in the tub, or try other natural methods. Option two is to break your water. Option three is to start Pitocin,"* and so on. You and your family will decide what you desire to experience or not to experience in the progression of your labor.

This approach breaks down walls of resistance, especially for families transferring from birth centers or home births to the hospital. These families often fear losing autonomy and being subjected to unwanted medicalization of their birth experience. I sit at the bedside and begin my introduction when I meet them. I ask, *"Tell me what is most important to you and your family in your birth experience. How can I help you achieve your desired birth while keeping you and your family safe?"*

Sandy's Story

Sandy arrived at the hospital and was taken into my care from a birth center after pushing for over four hours. She was accompanied by her husband, sister, and doula. Sandy, a vibrant 26-year-old with tattoos covering her body, was in visible pain. Her husband, equally tattooed and muscular, stood protectively between us, declaring, *"No C-section; we did not come here to be told we had to have a C-section. We did come for rest and more time."*

I sat on a stool at Sandy's eye level, softening the tension in the room. After introducing myself and explaining my approach, I asked, *"What are your goals, and how can I assist?"* Together, we discussed her pregnancy journey. Sandy requested an epidural and two hours of rest. Afterward, I proposed options: continuing to push or transitioning to a C-section if there was no progress. I expressed considerable safety concerns, major risk of infection, hemorrhage, and pelvic floor dysfunction, but the family insisted on pushing. Four hours later, with no movement and increasing swelling of the baby's head, I pleaded for a safe transition to a C-section.

At this point, the family was saddened and dismayed by the final recommendation. Sandy's twin sister revealed she had also required C-sections, raising the possibility of genetic factors at play. Moreover, Dad expressed how strong he knows his wife to be. She is a palate and yoga instructor. She was squatting 180 lbs through the early part of the third trimester. Even more revealing of

Sandy's resolve, she has had to retrain herself to walk after a horse injury that fractured her pelvis at age 16. After one year of intensive rehabilitation, she is now an excellent warrior who can't push out a baby. Dad, sister, and Sandy were all very disappointed.

With these new revelations, I reassessed the situation. I now better understand why and how we found ourselves in this position. Sandy's story underscores the importance of collaboration, patience, and deep listening to patients' needs.

April's Resolve

April, a 29-year-old Islander, came to my clinic in tears. I hadn't even introduced myself or my philosophy of care. This was her fifth pregnancy. Her first baby was breech, leading to a necessary C-section. Her subsequent pregnancies followed a pattern of denied opportunities for trial of labor, culminating in repeat C-sections. April was determined to attempt a vaginal birth after a cesarean (VBAC) but had faced resistance and potential medical bullying.

I began by explaining the American College of Obstetricians and Gynecologists (ACOG) guidelines for VBAC:

1. **Emergency Cesarean Capability:** Facilities must be equipped for immediate surgical intervention.
2. **On-Site Surgical and Anesthesia Personnel:** Resources should be readily available.

3. **Informed Consent:** Patients must fully understand the risks and benefits.

4. **Resource Considerations:** Providers should discuss limitations if resources are not available.

I outlined the risks: uterine rupture, placental abruption, and the potential for emergency C-sections with significant complications. I explained in detail, with some graphic communication, that I would transition to life-saving maneuvers in an emergency. I would move so quickly that I could injure organs that require additional surgeries to get her back to normal. She might need to wear an ostomy bag if her bowels were injured or experienced an occurrence of excessive blood loss, leading to a hysterectomy or admission to the ICU.

I expressed that I would prefer a scheduled C-section, as this is a high risk to me and my practice as well. Therefore, I will be bound to the hospital and her bedside until the baby is born, safe in her arms. I expressed to April, *"I cannot force you to have a C-section, but my recommendation today would be in line with the standard of care. I recommend a repeat C-section for your baby's safety. If you choose to go against that recommendation, I request you sign documentation against medical advice. And my focus would shift to making sure you remain safe."*

April's resolve was clear: *"I can do this. No one has given me the chance."* Her husband supported her, saying, *"This may be our last child, and I support my wife's decision."* Once again, I re-stated the risk to her husband specifically: *"Your risk of uterine rupture or placenta abruption could be as high as 20-30%, coupled with the risk of ICU admission, hysterectomy, and other major complications."*

While I could not endorse a plan outside standard guidelines, I committed to being present for her. *"Every time we meet, I will remind you of the risks and recommend a C-section,"* I said. *"If you proceed, you must stay on continuous monitoring, and in an emergency, you must trust my lead without hesitation."* April agreed.

The Bigger Picture

Patients like April and Sandy highlight the tension between medical guidelines and patient autonomy. While safety remains paramount, these experiences emphasize the need for respect, compassion, and shared decision-making. After interactions with other providers, I have had patients who have received communications such as, "Absolutely not, you will do this my way," or "I am the doctor; you listen to me, " *etc."* As a result, they chose to labor in a hotel next to the hospital in hopes that if urgency arose, they would be close enough to receive care. Others opt for Midwives to perform VBAC after two C-sections on an unproven pelvis or to assist with a breech birth with mono-dizygotic twins at home.

Sandy was poorly educated on her chances to deliver vaginally. Her delivery team did not listen to what the family provided about their history. And though they were supported in their attempt for vaginal delivery, they were allowed to be in jeopardy to achieve this autonomy.

Ultimately, April's journey was not just about delivering a baby; it was about reclaiming autonomy. She chose me as her provider because I respected her right to make informed decisions (good or bad). In supporting her, I reaffirmed my commitment to safe and empowering care. It is her body, her baby, and her choice—and my role is to provide skilled, compassionate care to achieve the best possible outcome.

Chapter 4

Restoring Trust in Birth: The Power of Informed Consent and Patient Autonomy

Informed Trust

During patient introductions, one of my most vivid memories was meeting a young woman named Jessica, who cried uncontrollably for nearly 30 minutes. Her pain and anguish were palpable, as though she were reliving a traumatic event. Jessica had been in counseling for months, yet her despair remained evident. She wasn't pregnant but was considering a second pregnancy after what she described as a disastrous birth experience.

Jessica shared that she had felt a connection with her doctor throughout her first pregnancy. However, the day she arrived at the hospital in labor, things took a tragic turn. Laboring unmedicated at 3 a.m., she declined the epidural her doctor had recommended. When the doctor arrived at 6 a.m., she entered the room, asked for a tool resembling a crochet hook (an amnio hook), opened her legs, and broke her bag of water. The umbilical cord immediately fell between her legs. A cord prolapses. All of this was done without saying a single word to her. There was no informed consent. The next thing she knew, she was being rushed to the operating room, put under general anesthesia, and awoke to find her baby in a warmer beside her.

Jessica and her husband were not present for the birth of their child. She had no joyous memories of that day, only trauma. She confessed she had struggled to bond with her baby despite months of counseling and felt lost in the aftermath of her experience. The person she trusted the most in that environment had provided the least safety.

In my practice, I protect the patient's autonomy and emphasize the importance of informed consent. I explicitly outline that I will not do anything to you without their knowledge or agreement. Yet, I also prepare them for moments of urgency, trusting that they will understand if full communication isn't possible in such situations. But a discussion should occur in routine procedures like breaking the bag of water to progress labor. Patients deserve to have autonomy in their care.

In Jessica's case, the conversation could have been as simple as:

"Jessica, your baby and labor are progressing well. There's no urgency, but at this time, you have options. Option one: do nothing and let your body continue to labor naturally. Option two: speed things up by breaking the bag of water or starting Pitocin to make the contractions stronger and closer together."

I would then explain the pros and cons of each option:

1. Waiting: This allows natural progression but may take longer. The advantage is continuing without interventions like enabling mobility and intermittent monitoring. Strategies like walking, using a birth ball, or getting in a tub could help.

2. Pitocin: This medicine, though sometimes maligned, is one of the most valuable tools in Obstetrics. Properly used, More than 90% of those who chose Pitocin will have zero complications. Mismanagement, however, can lead to complications like uterine atony or postpartum hemorrhage. Patients must know they're in control; Pitocin should never be increased without their consent. They can request adjustments or discontinuation anytime, as long as safety allows. Our job is to support you through this, not force this upon you.

3. Breaking the Bag of Water: This can accelerate labor by applying the baby's head directly to the cervix, but often increases the intensity of labor pains. It's a point of no return, as the action cannot be undone. Patients must weigh the benefits and risks carefully. Breaking the bag does NOT initiate a time clock, meaning delivery must occur within 24–48 hours. This is poor communication that leads to fear and medical bullying.

This approach, centered on informed consent, epitomizes modern medicine's strengths. However, time constraints often hinder thorough communication, especially in busy clinics with brief appointments. This imbalance sometimes leads to patients feeling rushed or unheard, a failing of the system that prioritizes efficiency over empathy.

Sandy's Story Continues

After extensive discussions outlining the risks, benefits, and alternatives, Sandy and her husband agreed to proceed with a C-section. Intraoperatively, her entire pelvis was bruised from prolonged labor and pushing. Postoperatively, Sandy experienced a foot drop due to a pelvic hematoma compressing a nerve, requiring extended physical therapy. Although the couple was grateful for the care, the experience left them with lingering PTSD and reluctance to pursue future pregnancies. They later expressed that had they been fully informed earlier, they would have opted for a C-section sooner, potentially avoiding much of the trauma.

Reflection

Stories like Jessica's and Sandy's highlight the critical need for clear communication and patient empowerment. While the constraints of modern healthcare often challenge this ideal, the principle remains unchanged: patients deserve to understand their options and make informed decisions about their care. As providers, we must prioritize these conversations, ensuring every patient feels heard, respected, and supported in their journey toward safe and fulfilling birth experiences.

Chapter 5

Reclaiming Birth: Addressing Trauma and Restoring Autonomy in Maternity Care

Unlike other medical specialties, patients choose their Obstetrician based on the quality of care and the experience they wish to have. Patients often drive hours from their homes to deliver with a provider known for this dual ability. In contrast, emergency care is sought at the nearest facility, regardless of the provider's reputation. What drives this deliberate search for care? It is the widespread trauma, or Post Traumatic Stress Disorder (PTSD), ingrained in our maternity care system. Patients live not only in their own stories, like Salima or Jessica, but also in the experiences of their family and friends.

Nearly every day, during intake with a new patient, I hear stories of trauma suffered by others as justification for their choices—whether avoiding specific procedures or traveling great distances from places like Flagstaff, Bullhead City, Arizona, Cottonwood, Tucson, Ohio, Florida, Canada, and even Great Britain. This PTSD drives individuals to seek out care providers who can offer both healing and recovery. This very pursuit is what fuels my passion for this work.

It was brought into sharp focus when I overheard a chief resident say to a junior resident: *"No, we can't do this to her. We are part of the problem! Pre-eclampsia doesn't automatically mean a C-section. We must give her a chance if her labs and blood pressure remain stable. Keep pushing on. We have to stop inflicting trauma on these patients and practice good medicine."* I then realized the work I was doing was translational, that not only was I helping patients, but I was also helping doctors. I am assisting in the practice of Obstetrics. The medical assault on patients must end.

Carla's Autonomy Denied

One of the patients who epitomized this issue was Carla. At 44 years old, she was referred to me by MFM at 30 weeks pregnant, having had minimal prenatal care. Carla's BMI exceeded 50, with most of the weight concentrated centrally. Her first pregnancy had ended in a C-section because her doctor convinced her it was the safest option for her and her baby, given her size (you may recall this same theme with Jennifer). This marked the start of a cascade of events. She returned to her provider, now four C-sections later, all with the same provider. Carla described her OB as her savior, someone she trusted implicitly for having delivered her children safely. She held the provider in high esteem, and by all means, the provider did nothing wrong. The provider used their knowledge and preferences to dictate a care plan and path that has led to four seemingly uncomplicated births (c-sections).

Yet, Carla was sitting in front of me, emotionally torn. Her husband's anger and frustration were palpable as he recounted how their trusted OB had dismissed them from his practice, deeming her *"too high risk"* after a difficult fourth C-section. Carla, now 44 years old, has had an increased BMI since her younger years. Furthermore, the notes from her doctor suggest the abdomen was full of scar tissue. The doctor went to his team of well-trained providers and their partners, and unanimously, they chose to excuse Carla from the practice. As a collaborative group, they would not take the liability of her fifth C-section at 44 years old.

Carla had approached five other practices, all of which had refused to care for her. And why should they now accept her if her provider had excused her? What moral obligation did these other practices have to Carla if her own provider chose to dismiss her? My anger was unmatched at that moment, and I shed tears for Carla. I felt her trauma, and I felt her husband's distrust of the medical system, which feared for his wife's health while shouldering the burden of their family's future. They had four children and a farm to run. Carla had lost her autonomy years ago, never fully informed of the gravity of each decision made for her, not by her.

Informed Consent

Jessica's case was another heartbreaking example. Her emergency C-section followed an assault during labor. The lack of proper consent and counseling compounded her trauma. Had she been an active participant in her care decisions, she might have felt some sense of urgency to accept an artificial rupture of membranes (AROM), and clinical outcomes would have remained unchanged. Jessica might have requested not to have her membranes ruptured at that time. As providers, we are obligated to inform our patients of the options and all potential outcomes. If URGENCY is not present, allowing for questions and answers ultimately enables the patient and family to decide on the appropriate care plan. It's her body, and it's her baby.

The PTSD of birth doesn't just affect patients; it affects the entire family—Carla's and Jessica's husbands, to say the least. It also impacts providers, nurses, and staff. The weight of postpartum hemorrhages, neonatal deaths, and maternal mortality—extreme cases I have thankfully not encountered—leaves a mark. Even when best practices are followed, trauma can still result.

Carla's and Jessica's providers did what more than 85% of providers would have done. In the court of law, they performed above the standard of care, not just in offering the C-section for obesity, but in discharging them from the practice. The doctor did nothing wrong, yet morally, they abandoned a patient needing their care.

Georgiana's Story

Several years ago, Georgiana walked into my office, a 27-year-old. This was their very first pregnancy, and as a couple, they were as excited as most. Georgiana had several challenges in the pregnancy. She is obese with a BMI around 50. She had diabetes and hypertension. She and her partner transferred to my practice at 20 weeks because the few providers she saw explicitly spoke of a C-section immediately after meeting. They told her monitoring would be hard, and her baby would be too big because of the diabetes.

She was told, *"You would rather have a controlled C-section in the case of urgency, so just plan for a C-section from the start."* But she and her partner did not want a C-section.

I explained that while the concerns mentioned were valid, she could also come in, labor, and deliver without complication. She should be given the opportunity for a vaginal birth. I also emphasized that a C-section is not a benign procedure; it carries additional risks, such as poor wound healing due to her medical conditions. Yet, if an emergency C-section were needed, it would not be easy with her BMI. A fast surgery would have a higher risk of injury to her and the baby. Such a case might require C-sections in the future. After discussing her options, she chose to attempt a vaginal birth.

The anxiety surrounding her labor was palpable. When she arrived at the labor and delivery unit, I held a team huddle with the charge nurse, residents, and her assigned nurse. I stated:

"The patient has been informed of the risks and benefits and consented to a C-section. Due to her body habitus, exams should be limited to those necessary for clinical indications, as uterine infection could increase the likelihood of a C-section. Notify me of any fetal heart rate changes, but under limited circumstances are we rushing to the OR there must be a definitive case of fetal bradycardia or a progressively worsening fetal tracing. We will tolerate category II tracings if there is reactivity and overall good fetal reserve."

Her labor lasted two days, with occasional category II variables and a rare late deceleration. She was checked only three times throughout labor. Ultimately, she progressed to full dilation, pushed for five minutes, and delivered successfully.

Had she labored elsewhere, she likely would have undergone a medically unnecessary C-section—one that would have been justifiable by clinical guidelines but avoidable in reality. As we discuss overall general health- vaginal birth remains the healthiest way to deliver a baby. Moreover, this exemplifies Her Body, Her Baby- where maternal experience is consider on par with fetal outcome. Georgiana's voice were heard in her care.

Jennifer's Determination

Her story stood out as a lesson in perseverance. Pregnant with natural triplets—two mono-mono and one di—Jennifer, like any other family, was in shock. Clinic visit after clinic visit occurred until reality set in, and she met with a high-risk specialist. Multiple specialists had advised Jennifer to terminate the twins to save the singleton. Each consultation was grim, emphasizing doom and shattering her faith and hope. Then, she found Dr. Everett MFM, who referred her to me as the delivering provider. Together, we mapped out a plan: extended hospitalization, frequent monitoring, and the understanding that her babies wouldn't go past 32 weeks. Jennifer carried her triplets to 32 weeks, delivering healthy babies under our care. Yet, she later confided her daily trauma—living in constant fear of bad news with every non-stress test or ultrasound evaluation.

As providers, I now realize we build that fear of a negative outcome. We focus so heavily on the negative what-ifs and often forget that those living in that space suffer. So, what if it goes well? What if we get to 32 weeks? What about the words of encouragement that state, *"I am here and will be here in the time of need. I can't guarantee the outcome, but I will be with you every step of the way. This is why I became a doctor, this is why I chose OB, and this is why I am here to help and honor your family's wishes and desires in this setting as long as you are safe."*

Brittney's Experience

Brittney was another patient who taught me to see birth through a different lens. As beautiful as birth is for so many, for others it can be traumatic. Brittney, pregnant at 27 weeks, her membranes ruptured. At the realization of the potential 7 weeks in the hospital, realizing the baby would spend weeks in NICU, Brittney would not be able to repeat her last birth. Brittney delivered her first baby in the hospital with an Ob/gyn, Her second baby was a free birth at home in her closet with the family dog being the first to bless the experience. This time, Brittney had hoped for a home birth with a Midwife team to yield more structure but considerably less than the hospital birth. Despite her fears, we developed a plan to prolong the pregnancy. Brittney's past experiences shaped her wishes: minimal interventions and autonomy in delivery. However, complications arose, necessitating a C-section. For Brittney, the procedure symbolized a ritualistic *"satanic"* ordeal—a stark contrast to the empowering birth she desired. Her description of masked individuals, bright lights, unfamiliar chants (medical terminology), sharp knives, and repeated words in a say once, cutting the baby from the mother's belly and holding the baby high in the sky for ceremonial praise. This idea forever changed how I view surgical births.

Reflection

This chapter of my career has instilled a profound understanding of the human element in Obstetrics. ACOG emphasizes individualized care plans. Attending an ABC Board Review course underscored this for me. We must adjust plans to meet the unique needs of each patient, recognizing the risks of trauma inherent in one-size-fits-all approaches. Whether through personalized prenatal care, tailored postpartum support, or individualized birth plans, our role is to restore autonomy and humanity in childbirth.

Ultimately, it's her body, her baby, and as long as she is safe, her voice must lead the way.

Chapter 6

Defying Doubts: A Journey in Patient-Centered Obstetric Care

I was closing out my four long years of residency, ultimately culminating in seven intensive years of higher medical education training. I had become board-eligible in both Family Medicine, Obstetrics, and Gynecology. Now a father of two young children, both under six, and with my wife working grueling weekend night shifts, the responsibility of finding a job and beginning our next chapter fell squarely on my shoulders. Yet, I was adrift, uncertain of where to go or what to do.

Then, my wife mentioned that one of the Attending Physicians on the unit, Dr. McGill, was discussing retirement. He had a thriving private practice, and so I inquired. As the months flew by and graduation loomed closer, I made a decision. I would open my practice under Dr. McGill's guidance and mentorship. I was exhilarated. The news spread quickly, and the nursing staff at my base hospital were thrilled to hear I was staying local to support Dr. McGill's patients. Premier Ob/Gyn LLC was founded.

One evening, as I was leaving the hospital, Dr. Okefee and Dr. Christian pulled me aside. Their conversation was unexpected and unsettling. Dr. Okefee questioned my decision to enter private practice as a male and minority provider in the greater Phoenix area, suggesting the challenges ahead would be insurmountable. He doubted whether Dr. McGill's loyal patient base would transfer to me once McGill retired. He even raised concerns about my ability to support my young family. Dr. Christian, echoing the sentiment mockingly, joked that his practice would get busier as my patients either transferred or were referred out. I felt cornered and attacked, but their doubts only fueled my determination to succeed.

Dr. McGill's mentorship was invaluable. His civil and individualized approach to patient care was groundbreaking. He embraced alternative strategies to achieve the best outcomes, empowering patients to make informed decisions. His patients were allowed to labor without rigid time constraints, consider breech births, or pursue unmedicated VBACs under careful monitoring. He taught me hands-on skills like breech extractions and forceps-assisted deliveries. Through association, my practice began to grow.

In the meantime, my wife decided to leave her nursing role in labor and delivery to pursue Midwifery school. After two years of hard work, she graduated. When Midwifery jobs proved scarce, I invited her to join my practice, bringing the Midwifery model of care into our collaborative approach. Together, we transformed

Premier OB-GYN into what it represents today, blending personalized care, Dr. McGill's progressive methods, and my wife's expertise to offer something unique.

Our practice became a magnet for patients seeking individualized care. We worked with birth centers, advocacy groups, and VBAC supporters like ICAN. One such patient was April. She poured her heart out, sharing her experiences of feeling dismissed and harmed by the healthcare system. Despite having four previous C-sections, she was resolute: she wanted a vaginal birth.

April knew the scrutiny she'd face from the medical community but remained steadfast. Together, we reviewed the risks and care standards as ACOG recommended. April understood the challenges and signed informed consent forms acknowledging the risks. On the day of her labor, the hospital atmosphere was tense, filled with whispers and judgment. The background noise was deafening: *"Is he really going to let her do this?" "This isn't safe." "What's wrong with her? Doesn't she care about her baby?"*

I called a multidisciplinary meeting, gathering the charge nurse, anesthesia team, residents, and others. I laid out April's care plan and emphasized that while I did not endorse her decisions, I was committed to providing her with safe, professional care. My role was to ensure that, as long as she and her baby were safe, she had the autonomy to make her own choices. Within four hours, April delivered a healthy nine-pound baby vaginally with no complications.

April's case reaffirmed my belief in respecting patient autonomy. Supporting their choices does not equate to agreement; yet care demands professionalism and empathy.

Denise's Resolute Autonomy

Another example is Denise, who came to my practice at 38 weeks and five days. It is always peculiar when someone maintains care with their provider until the week before delivery and then switches. The only reason for this is often provider neglect. Denise had experienced an uncomplicated pregnancy, but her baby was measuring large. She was sent to Maternal-Fetal Medicine for an ultrasound, which estimated the fetal weight at 10 lbs. 4 oz. MFM recommended delivery via C-section at 39 weeks.

Despite expressing her desire for a vaginal birth, MFM proceeded to schedule a primary C-section. Angry and feeling disregarded, Denise entered my office for a consultation. Denise again expressed her strong desire for a natural birth. I reviewed the details and the data, breaking down the situation using the SBAR approach.

S - Situation

- Term pregnancy

- Macrosomia – Estimated fetal weight +/- 350 to 440 grams (1 lb)
- Maternal desire for natural birth (autonomy)

B - Background

- Unproven pelvis
- Large babies increase the risk of shoulder dystocia, which could lead to major fetal injury or even fetal death.

A - Alternatives

- Primary C-section (standard of care)
- Come in laboring, but if labor progression falls off the labor curve, transition to a C-section for safety.

R - Recommendations:

The data on macrosomia is just that—data. However, we need to use it to guide decisions that prioritize safety.

For every controversial complicated decision, it always comes down to this discussion about the two different family's consent scenarios:

- **Two Patient Consent Scenarios:**

I. Patient 1: *"Doctor, I have worked nine months to have a healthy baby and family. I will endure whatever I need to ensure my baby is okay."* For this family, the recommendation would be to follow MFM's advice and proceed with the C-section despite their personal preferences.

II. Patient 2: *"Doctor, if I endure unnecessary trauma, I don't know if I'll be okay. The psychological impact could deeply affect me, my newborn, and my family. I will transition to your recommend care plan but only after I do all that I can first. Can I have a chance to try, I must know deep down that I gave it my all."* For this situation, the clear recommendation would be to attempt a vaginal birth, with the understanding that any concerns during labor would necessitate a timely transition to a C-section to avoid injury or trauma.

Denise had just one visit with me, but we all agreed that the plan would transition for safety if any concerns arose during labor. At 39 weeks, Denise did not show up for her scheduled C-section. At 39 weeks and five days, I received a text from Denise saying she was in labor and heading to the hospital. I agreed to meet her there.

Twenty minutes later, she beat me to the hospital. As she crossed the OB triage door, she screamed, *"I need to push!"* Denise delivered a 10 lbs. 4 oz baby boy unmedicated and without a tear within minutes of arriving at the hospital. Yet, had she followed MFM's recommendations, she would have undergone an unnecessary C-section. Furthermore, the implications of that decision could have been significant, potentially relegating her to additional C-sections in future pregnancies, depending on where she received care.

Empowered Choice

In all my years as a medical practitioner, no patient challenged these principles more than Catherine. Catherine, a 25-year-old woman with a BMI of 50, drove four hours from Bullhead City to see me. She had experienced coercion during her previous labor, feeling pressured into a C-section after stalling at six centimeters. Starting a new pregnancy, she was resolute in her desire for a VBAC.

From the start, I introduced Catherine to my *"five Ps"* for successful vaginal delivery:

1. **Power:** The effectiveness of uterine contractions and maternal pushing.

2. **Pelvis:** The maternal pelvis's adequacy to allow passage of the fetus.

3. **Passenger:** The fetus's size, position, and presentation.

4. **Psych:** The psychological readiness and support systems of the birthing person.

5. **Provider**: The healthcare providers role is to foster trust and manage complications.

At 34 weeks and three days, Catherine's water broke. She arrived at OB triage with meconium-stained fluid and irregular contractions. An ultrasound revealed the baby was oblique. Despite the risks—PPROM, fetal growth restriction, and her BMI (50)—Catherine declined a C-section and insisted on continuing her VBAC plan. Over the next few days, the baby's position fluctuated between cephalic and breech, necessitating repeated discussions about risks and options. MFM and Hospital Risk Management Team were asked to come to the bedside and counsel Catherine on her decisions. The conclusion was safety.

Each shift change brought new frustrations from the care team, but I reminded everyone that Catherine's autonomy was paramount as long as she and the baby remained stable. By the fifth day, after multiple assessments and attempts to induce labor safely, Catherine finally requested a repeat C-section. The procedure was uncomplicated, and both mother and baby went home healthy.

In her postpartum visit, Catherine expressed immense gratitude. We hugged and celebrated the shared journey of perseverance and trust.

It's her baby. It's her body. Patients deserve a voice in their care as long as safety is maintained.

These stories reflect the core of my practice: respecting patient autonomy while ensuring safety. Whether it was April's high-risk VBAC, Denise's trust in her instincts, or Catherine's perseverance, each woman reminded me that care isn't just clinical—it's deeply personal. When we listen, support, and stand beside our patients, we don't just deliver babies—we help deliver trust, dignity, and lasting change in how care is given.

Chapter 7

Autonomy in Maternity Care: Provider Roles and Challenges

Birth Objectives By Provider

Subject/Item	LPM/CPM	CNM	Private practice MD	Academic MD	corporate MD	HospitalistMD
safe baby	xx	xxx	xxxx	xxxx	xxxx	xxxx
safe mom	xxx	xxxx	xxxx	xxx	xxxx	xxxx
maternal-fetal connection	xxx	xxx	xx	xx	x	
mind and body healing	xxx	xxxx	xx	x		
autonomy	xxx	xxxx	xx	x		
PTSD and trauma	xxx	xxx	x			
empowering women	xxx	xxxx	x			

The comparative framework of birth objectives highlights how each provider's position or training intersects with autonomy in maternity care. Autonomy, or the ability of birthing individuals to make informed decisions about their care, remains a central yet variably prioritized element in childbirth work. The table reflects differing emphasis on autonomy among Licensed Professional Midwives and Certified Professional Midwives (LPM and CPM), MidwivesCertified Nurse Midwives (CNM), and various categories of Medical Doctors (MD), including Private Practice MDs, Academic MDs, Corporate MDs, and Hospitalist MDs. Each provider type brings unique challenges and strengths to promoting autonomy in maternity care, often influenced by their training, scope of practice, and institutional context.

Midwifery Models: Licensed Professional Midwives and Certified Professional Midwives (LPM and CPMs)

LPM and CPMs place a high emphasis on autonomy *("xxx"),* as their care models center on informed consent and individualized approaches. Their training and philosophy often prioritize shared decision-making, fostering a deep maternal-fetal connection, and empowering women. However, these Midwives typically operate in out-of-hospital settings, which can pose challenges when emergencies arise or when care transitions to hospital-based providers with differing priorities. Despite these hurdles, the Midwifery model of care remains a cornerstone for autonomy-driven practices.

MidwivesCertified Nurse Midwives (CNMs)

CNMs exhibit the strongest support for autonomy *("xxxx"),* reflecting their integration of evidence-based practice with holistic care. They often practice in hospitals and birthing centers, giving them the flexibility to combine natural childbirth principles with medical interventions when necessary. CNMs' advanced nursing background equips them to navigate institutional constraints while advocating for patient-centered care. Nevertheless, systemic barriers—such as hospital policies or hierarchical dynamics with physicians—can sometimes limit their ability to support autonomous decision-making fully.

Medical Doctors: A Spectrum of Autonomy Support

Private Practice MDs

Private Practice MDs show moderate emphasis on autonomy *("xx").* Their training in Obstetrics often emphasizes clinical safety and adherence to standardized protocols, which may inadvertently constrain patient choices. However, the private practice setting can allow for more personalized care, providing opportunities to discuss options in depth. Balancing medical expertise with patient preferences remains a challenge for these providers, particularly when managing complex or high-risk pregnancies.

Academic MDs

Academic MDs also prioritize autonomy at a moderate level *("xx")*. Their dual roles as educators and practitioners often position them at the forefront of evidence-based practices, which can enhance shared decision-making. However, the demands of teaching, research, and institutional protocols can limit their capacity to engage deeply with individual preferences. This tension between academic responsibilities and patient-centered care is a notable challenge in this group.

Corporate MDs

Corporate MDs place minimal emphasis on autonomy *("x")*, reflecting the efficiency-driven and standardized nature of care in corporate healthcare settings. These providers often work within systems prioritizing cost-effectiveness and streamlined protocols, which may restrict individualized care. While corporate models can enhance access to services, the trade-off often comes at the expense of patient autonomy, leaving limited room for personalized decision-making.

Hospitalist MDs

Hospitalist MDs, who provide acute care within hospital settings, also demonstrate minimal emphasis on autonomy *("x")*. Their role focuses on immediate clinical needs, often under time and resource constraints. This environment can make it challenging to engage in nuanced discussions about patient preferences, particularly during emergencies. Despite these limitations, hospitalist MDs play a crucial role in ensuring safety and addressing urgent medical concerns, often collaborating with other providers to support patient-centered care when feasible.

Challenges in Promoting Autonomy in Birth Work

1. **Systemic Constraints:** Institutional policies, hierarchical dynamics, and efficiency pressures can limit providers' ability to support autonomy fully.

2. **Provider Training:** The emphasis on clinical safety in medical education often overshadows training in shared decision-making and patient advocacy, particularly for MDs.

3. **Risk Perception:** Differing attitudes toward risk influence how providers balance autonomy with safety. Midwives may prioritize empowering choices, while MDs may lean toward intervention to mitigate perceived risks.

4. **Communication Barriers:** In multidisciplinary settings, divergent philosophies and practices can hinder effective collaboration, impacting the consistent support of autonomy.

5. **Resource Limitations:** Time constraints, staffing shortages, and administrative burdens can restrict the depth of patient-provider discussions about care options.

The intersection of provider roles, training, and institutional contexts significantly shapes how autonomy is prioritized in maternity care. Midwives (LPM, CPMs, and CNMs) emerge as leaders in fostering autonomy, emphasizing individualized care and empowerment. In contrast, MDs, particularly those in corporate or hospitalist roles, often face systemic and institutional challenges that limit their capacity to support autonomous decision-making fully. Addressing these disparities requires systemic changes, including better integrating holistic principles in medical training, improved interdisciplinary collaboration, and patient-centered policy reforms. By navigating these challenges, maternity care can better align with birthing individuals diverse needs and preference s, ensuring both safety and autonomy in one of life's most transformative experiences.

Reflections on Communication and Autonomy-Challenges in Communication

Throughout my training, I have been taught that there are various ways to communicate with patients. I had initially adopted these methods of communication and attempted to persuade patients into and out of care plans. The goal always is and was to obtain confidence in the patients so that you, the provider, can influence patient care. Over the years, I have learned this form and communicated that certain practices interfere with a more autonomous approach to care. Despite the strong stance of organizations like ACOG on individualized care, some common statements contradict these principles:

- ***"I Am the Expert":*** This approach suggests providers should communicate best practices without allowing patients to question or second-guess their guidance. The analogy often given is: *"You wouldn't tell your car mechanic how to do their job; similarly, patients shouldn't question their doctor."* Such communication clearly undermines autonomy and establishes an authoritarian dynamic.

A Case in Point: Individualized Care vs. Authoritarian Communication

I recall a conversation with an engineering family. When I introduced my care philosophy, the father said, *"Doctor, but you are the expert."* I replied, *"In my expertise, I recognize that each family and individual is uniquely different. Working on a Toyota Corolla engine means every engine is the same, but no two patients are identical. The best care adjusts to meet each circumstance."* This approach resonated with them, highlighting how empowering communication fosters trust and autonomy.

Risk-Focused Narratives

Another pervasive statement is, ***"All That Matters Is a Healthy Baby."*** This was recently conveyed during a fetal strip review. A provider noted, *"In the end, we're judged on the baby's outcome."* This mindset often drives early escalation to interventions like C-sections, as delays are harshly criticized if the baby is harmed. While safety is paramount, framing discussions solely around outcomes for the baby overlooks the broader context of maternal well-being and informed consent.

Relational Persuasion: "If You Were My Family..."

Statements like, ***"If You Were My Family Member, This Is What I'd Recommend,"*** are often used to soften authoritative communication. While this can build rapport, it can also manipulate patients into decisions aligned with the provider's preferences rather than genuinely informed choices. For example, when a patient presented with anxiety after a prior full-term demise, her tears reflected a deep desire to avoid past trauma. Instead of being offered nuanced options for her care, she was gently but firmly persuaded toward the provider's preferred course of action by the use of the words *"I would tell my wife or family the same."*

A Better Approach: Presenting Options

Providing clear, informed options empowers patients. For the above case, the same patient with the term demise, these might include:

1. **Higher-Level Monitoring:** Remaining in the hospital for ongoing care and rapid response if concerns arise; however, the downsides include the cost of hospitalization and an extended length of stay.

2. **Routine Care at Home:** Returning for regular evaluations and understanding the low risk based on current assessments. Though there are no guarantees, trust that we can transition and escalate care quickly if needed from home.

3. **Immediate Delivery:** Acknowledging the risks of prematurity, including the potential need for a prolonged hospital stay and rare but not uncommon complications for the baby, while also aligning with the patient's mental health priorities.

Such approaches avoid paternalistic communication and center on the patient's autonomy, ensuring care aligns with medical safety and individual preferences.

Reflection

This balance between clinical expertise and patient-centered care is no different for Salima, Jessica, April, or Habid. By respecting autonomy and fostering collaboration, we can honor the unique journeys of all birthing individuals.

In maternity care, autonomy is essential, but its support varies across providers. Midwives, particularly LPMs, CPMs, and CNMs, emphasize informed choice, emotional support, and empowerment, while many MDs, especially in corporate or hospital settings, face systemic constraints that can limit autonomy. Through my own experience, I've learned that genuine care involves guiding patients and respecting their informed decision-making. Communication that empowers (informs the patient fully without excessive bias), rather than persuades, fosters trust and aligns care with the patient's needs and values. It's about presenting options, acknowledging risks, and honoring each individual's unique journey.

Chapter 8

Balancing Autonomy and Care in Maternal Medicine

Providing maternal care is one of medicines most rewarding yet complex roles. It demands a unique balance: caring for two patients simultaneously—the mother and her baby. Unlike other medical specialties, where the focus is often singular, maternity care requires navigating the intertwined well-being of both.

The baby, unable to advocate for itself, relies entirely on clinical expertise, monitoring, and intuition. Meanwhile, the mother brings her voice—expressing preferences, emotions, and fears, often amplified by supportive family members. This dynamic creates a delicate interplay of objective medical care and deeply personal human experiences.

Achieving this balance requires more than medical expertise. It demands empathy, trust, and collaborative decision-making between all vested individuals (patient, family, provider, nurses, etc)- even the unborn baby. It means placing the mother's desires and experiences at the heart of care while ensuring the safety of both lives she carries.

Two patients. One goal. And yet, the paths to that goal can differ profoundly.

What About the Mother?

Two women—Habid and Denise—represent the essence of this challenge. Habid's decision to prioritize avoiding a high-risk surgery, even if it meant a devastating loss. Denise's determination to deliver her ten-pound, four-ounce baby vaginally to avoid the potential aftermath of a C-section. Their stories bring forward a critical question:

For too long, the weight of pregnancy and childbirth has leaned heavily on the baby's needs, often overshadowing the mother's autonomy, desires, and experience. But how do we honor both lives while providing the individualized care that ACOG advocates for?

When I meet my patients, my message is clear:

"I'm not here to tell you what to do or how to do it. I'm here to give you options so you can decide what's best for you, your body, and your baby, as long as you are safe."

And here's the truth: *"anything done to you without your consent is assault. My job is not to impose my will but to educate and empower you to make informed choices."*

These words challenge the traditional norms of training and practice. They provoke controversy and criticism, but acknowledge a simple, often overlooked truth: the mother's experience matters, therefore there is the freedom of choice in maternity cares.

Mary and Sophia: A Tale of Two Mothers

Six months apart, I had the honor of caring for Mary and Sophia—two women with similar circumstances but vastly different outcomes, due to the freedom of choice. Their stories illuminate the importance of centering care on the mother- patient centered care.

Mary's Story

Mary, a G3P1011, was a healthy young woman with a history of complicated C-sections for the first pregnancy, followed by a miscarriage. Now thrilled to be pregnant with the third, she came to me with a heavy heart after learning from her 19-week anatomy scan that her baby had hypoplastic right heart syndrome—a severe cardiac condition.

She was devastated.

Her first pregnancy had been traumatic. She'd hoped for a vaginal delivery but, after four hours of stalled labor, was rushed into a C-section. The recovery was brutal: wound infections, IV antibiotics, and home health visits. The idea of facing a similar recovery while caring for a critically ill newborn was unbearable.

Her current provider insisted on another C-section. Mary, terrified and overwhelmed, asked for my opinion. Her questions ranged from the necessity of genetic testing to the risks of attempting a VBAC with her baby's cardiac condition. How devastating is the diagnosis for the baby? Are there other options for me and the baby?

High-Risk Consents

When counseling patients facing complex decisions, I often explain that there are two types of families.

The first family says, *"Doctor, I will endure whatever I need to avoid any risk or complication for my baby. I will suffer; I'll accept a C-section (the proposed care plan, avoid medications, etc.), and the mom will work through the challenges it might present to her to avoid challenges or risk for the baby."*

The second family says, *"Doctor, if I go through immense suffering and struggle, I won't be in a good mental or physical state. This would be harmful to me and my family."* That family chooses to attempt alternative care plans, accepting that the baby might need additional care after birth. This family agrees to transition at real danger (risk to mom or baby), but the family needs to know they gave it a try before transitioning to the care plan proposed.

These distinctions matter profoundly in tailoring care plans that align with a familys values and priorities.

Mary chose the C-section. For her, prioritizing the outcome for the baby was essential in dealing with a challenging diagnosis. She wanted to ensure she would afford the best for her baby after delivery by avoiding any unnecessary risk. Mary was willing to endure another post c-section infection to avoid risk to the baby.

She had a wonderful C-section under the care of Dr. McGill and me. It was smooth, intentional, and everything she hoped it would be. Today, Mary's baby, Mighty Jack, thrives as a beacon of hope for many. Mary herself has become a counselor and advocate for families facing similar cardiac diagnoses, offering support to others navigating similar difficult decisions and emotions.

Sophia's Story

Sophia's situation bore some similarities to Mary's, but her circumstances and choices were vastly different. A little younger than Mary, Sophia was pregnant with her fourth child, having had three previous vaginal deliveries. She presented as a late transfer to our care, already well into her pregnancy and beyond the gestational age that would have allowed her controversial options.

Unlike Mary, Sophia had never been counseled on the indications for prenatal testing. When her anatomy scan at 22 weeks revealed the diagnosis of hypoplastic right heart, she was left with limited choices. The baby, though affected, was genetically normal.

Sophia lived in a remote rural area, caring for livestock and raising three young children. By the time we met, she had already formulated a care plan in her mind.

"I want to deliver vaginally," she said with quiet determination. *"Whatever happens, I don't want major interventions for the babys well -being. I don't want a c-section, or alternative specialcare in labor for the unborn baby. I want palliative care post delivery if needed."*

Sophia had resolved to follow her instincts and priorities, even knowing the challenges ahead. She was patient number two—a striking contrast to Mary, whose path had been clearer and more conventional. Sophia recognized that the physical and life challenges of multiple surgeries and interventions for her and the baby would yield extreme stress for her and her family. Who would manage the three other small children? Who would manage the farm when they spend weeks and months in the hospital for surgery and any medical setbacks?

These stories highlight the spectrum of decisions families must navigate when faced with high-risk pregnancies. Some prioritize their own health to ensure they can care for their baby; others prioritize the experience of birth or the baby's immediate needs, even if it means uncertainty or hardship later for the mother and the family.

Each choice is deeply personal, and as a provider, my role is not to dictate but to guide—to offer information, compassion, and unwavering support as families chart their course through the complexities of life and birth. Passing any form of judgement on either decision (Mary's or Sophia's) erodes the trust and confidence in modern medical system.

Despite hearing about success stories like Mighty Jack, Sophia chose palliative care. It was her way of preserving her family's stability and well-being.

Balancing Care: Autonomy and Informed Consent

These stories remind us that maternal care is not about imposing one s will but fostering informed, autonomous decision-making. The mother's voice matters.

In my practice, informed consent is a conversation, not a directive. It's about providing families with all the information: risks, benefits, alternatives, standards of care, and potential outcomes. It's about trust.

Mighty Jack thrives because Mary made the best decision for her. Sophia, too, made the best choice for her family, even if the outcome was different. Both stories reflect a truth we must never forget: True maternal care is not just about outcomes; it's about honoring every mother's journey, autonomy, and humanity. Outcomes matter, but we should accept even the unconventional outcome when there is an honest space for informed communication and all parties are at peace. One of my hardest deliveries, Johanna and Mark walked this tight rope- had informed communication with an outcome less than desired.

Resolution: Redefining Success in Maternal Care

Maternal care is not a formula—it is a relationship. It is not about perfect outcomes, but about meaningful, informed decisions made by empowered women in partnership with trusted clinicians.

Mary, Sophia, and countless others teach us this: success in maternal medicine must be redefined. It is not just about healthy babies and smooth deliveries. It is about respect. It is about choice. It is about honoring the mother's voice, even when her path diverges from our training or expectations.

As providers, our role is not to protect patients from hard decisions but to stand beside them as they make them—with honesty, compassion, and clarity. We do not own the outcomes, but we do bear responsibility for how those outcomes are reached: Was the patient heard? Was she given real options? Was she supported with dignity, not pressure?

Two patients. One goal. But many paths. The art of maternal medicine lies in walking those paths with humility—centering the mother, protecting the unborn, and ensuring that every decision is grounded in consent, not coercion.

When we do this well, even loss is met with peace. Even the hardest outcomes come with meaning. And birth, in all its forms, becomes not just a medical event—but a deeply human one.

Chapter 9

Setting the Stage for Autonomy in Labor

Johanna and Mark

Johanna and Mark arrived at the clinic united in pursuing a more natural and holistic second birth. Their first experience had been deeply challenging, marred by a cascade of interventions that ultimately culminated in a cesarean section. With their first child, Grant, conceived through IVF, Johanna's AMA (advanced maternal age) and gestational diabetes diagnosis had led their care team to push for induction. Intervention after intervention followed, leaving them with regret despite the joy of welcoming their son. For baby Harvey, they hoped for something different—something better.

When we first met, I began with an introduction that laid the foundation for their care: *"What I care about most is providing good care and a good experience. That means I'm not here to tell you what to do; I'm here to provide options so you can decide what's best for you, your baby, and your family, as long as it's safe. Anyone who does something to you without your consent is committing assault. My job is to educate you because educated individuals make educated decisions."*

As we delved into the details of their first labor, Johanna shared how her labor had stalled at 4cm for four hours. The baby had been in an OP (occiput posterior) position and was deemed unable to tolerate labor, leading to what was described as an *"emergency"* cesarean. Johanna's words were resolute: *"I want a healthy baby, but I definitely do not want another C-section under any circumstances."* Her statement resonated deeply, and I explained what would be required to achieve a vaginal birth.

I outlined the *"five Ps"* essential for a successful vaginal delivery:

1. **Power:** The ability to progress to full dilation and push effectively.
2. **Pelvis:** An adequate pelvis to allow the baby to pass through.
3. **Passenger:** A baby that participates by being well-positioned and tolerates labor without complications like a wrapped cord.
4. **Psyche:** The mental capacity and resolve to endure the marathon of labor.
5. **Provider:** A supportive provider who prioritizes patience and respects the birthing person's autonomy.

I emphasized that many providers view a healthy baby as the only outcome that matters, often pushing for C-sections at the first sign of fetal deceleration. In Johanna's case, her previous provider had deemed her high risk due to her age, IVF history, and weight, assuming she wouldn't want to *"risk"* her baby.

Mark asked, *"Do you think we're good candidates for a VBAC?"*

"Absolutely," I replied. *"I can't Monday morning quarterback, but your previous labor didn't progress enough to assess all the factors (the 5 P's). This time, we have an opportunity to approach things differently."*

We discussed the specifics of VBAC and TOLAC (trial of labor after cesarean). I explained my approach: being present when active labor was established, ensuring continuous monitoring, and having immediate care available in case of complications. I reviewed the risks and benefits, including the success rate of VBAC (70-80%) versus potential emergencies (2% risk of uterine rupture or placental abruption). 20-30% transition to C-section for the normal reasons. Therefore, I do not guarantee a vaginal birth rather I guarantee a different care – where you have a voice and will be heard. Together, we laid out a plan focused on autonomy and informed decision-making.

The pregnancy progressed smoothly. Johanna and Mark were proactive, implementing practices to encourage natural labor and avoid late-term complications. At 38 weeks and three days, they presented in active labor. Johanna was 4-5cm dilated, her membranes had ruptured, and their doula was by their side.

The Airplane Labor

When I met Johanna and Mark at the bedside, I began by laying out my rules of engagement. *"No one should do anything to you without your consent. We are here to offer you care, support, and options."* Once we established this understanding, they consented to a VBAC, and I ensured the necessary papers were signed for the hospital chart. I also answered all their questions thoroughly.

Mark, who was typically quiet during appointments, spoke up with conviction: *"We don't want another C-section."*

I explained their options clearly:

1. **Option 1: Do Nothing**
   This meant embracing natural labor methods: moving around, changing positions, using the tub, the birthing ball, or the myo-circuit.

2. **Option 2: Pitocin**
   I explained that we could start Pitocin at a low dose and increase it gradually up to a maximum of 20 milliunits, but only with Johanna's consent. I emphasized that she would be in

complete control of its use. *"No one will adjust the dose without asking you first. You can pause it, take a break, or maintain it at a level you're comfortable with,"* I reassured her.

After careful consideration, Johanna and Mark chose to pursue natural labor.

With the care plan established, I set the stage for labor by introducing them to my analogy of *"The Airplane Ride."*

"We're about to take off on this journey," I began. *"On this flight, I'll play two roles: first flight attendant and later the captain."*

I continued:
"As your flight attendant, I've just done my job by standing in the aisle and showing you all the safety features of this flight. I provided you with the options of labor, pain control, and the rules for a safe flight. But like any real flight, we might encounter turbulence."

Mark and Johanna listened intently as I explained the metaphor further.

"Turbulence in this context shows up in the fetal heart tracing when the baby's heart rate dips. If that happens, the flight attendants (care team) come to the room to ensure you and your baby are safe on the flight. They will turn and rotate you, hoping to get you out of turbulence. Like on a plane, an oxygen mask might fall from

the sky. We'll ask you to put oxygen on yourself first by taking measures to stabilize you and your baby. During turbulence, the seat belt sign comes on, and you must stay seated (remain in bed). Your fetal monitor is your seatbelt—this is how we ensure both of you are safe during the flight."

I paused to let them absorb the information before continuing.

"Finally, the captain speaks if turbulence occurs, just like on the airplane. That's me; I am the captain". Whether I'm physically here or in another part of the hospital, the crew is always in communication with me, and rest assured, I'm flying the plane."

I scanned their faces and continued,

"Now, we often fail to mention that turbulence tends to happen at two critical points during a flight: takeoff and landing.

Landing turbulence means we may need to land the plane quickly—sometimes gracefully and sometimes with a crash landing, like an assisted delivery or even a C-section.

Takeoff turbulence, however, is more concerning. We don't always know where we're headed. For example, if we're flying from Phoenix to San Francisco, we might just push through the bumps since it's a short flight. But if we're flying to Japan from Phoenix, which could take 14 to 18 hours, that's far too long to endure turbulence. In such cases, we may need to reroute for safety."

To my surprise, Mark lit up at the analogy. As a pilot himself, he was thrilled with the comparison and eagerly embraced his role as co-pilot for this journey.

Negative Results of Autonomy Misused

Johanna had chosen to *"do nothing"* and let her body take the lead. Several times, I returned to the room to check on her. Mark and Johanna, guided by their doula, were moving, swaying, and staying active, fully immersed in their labor process. I asked how they felt each time, reviewed the baby's tracing, and offered support. Each time, they politely declined any interventions.

Eight hours have passed since the last cervical exam. The baby was Category One, Johanna was afebrile, and there was no pressing medical need to intervene. At 16 hours, everything remained unchanged—steady progress but slow. They continued moving, laboring with determination.

By the 24 mark, the atmosphere shifted. Johanna's focus deepened; her moans became primal and raw. She requested an exam. Upon checking, I found she was fully dilated.

It was time to push.

The first hour was filled with effort and teamwork. We rotated positions, used tug-of-war with a sheet, tried the rebozo, and poured every ounce of energy into progress. Yet, after an hour, the baby had barely moved. Baby's heart rate remained stable, and Johanna felt great, buoyed by the encouragement of her doula and Mark. She wanted to keep going.

Another hour passed with the same outcome—minimal movement. Mom and baby were still holding steady, but the effort was starting to wane. Baby's heart rate began to lose some variability, though the beat-to-beat baseline remained reassuring. The baby's head was visible, just beyond the perineum.

I knew it was time to revisit our options.

"We can continue as we are, but there is some risk to the baby's well-being if we don't make progress soon," I explained. *"Alternatively, we can consider an assisted delivery with the vacuum or transition to a cesarean."* I outlined the risks and benefits of each option in detail, emphasizing the importance of preserving Johanna's pelvic floor and ensuring the baby's safety.

Johanna was tired—hot, naked, and visibly drained—but the doula was relentless in her encouragement. *"You've come so far,"* she told Johanna. *"This is your moment. Power up and push this baby out."* She repeatedly fed Johanna honey sticks, chanting, "You've got this!".

Johanna declined intervention. *"I'll push for 30 more minutes,"* she said. *"Then maybe I'll ask for help."*

Thirty minutes came and went. Still, there was no additional progress. I revisited the risks, reminding them of potential complications: pelvic floor dysfunction for Johanna, infection for the baby, and the possibility of NICU monitoring after birth. I also reiterated the risks of an assisted delivery: tearing, jaundice—but those risks paled in comparison to continuing without action.

The doula remained firm. *"You've got this!"* she cheered. The room echoed with chants of encouragement.

At this point, everyone was hitting their limits, especially the doula. She excused herself, explaining she could no longer extend herself in Johanna's care. My Jaw dropped!

When the door closed behind her, Johanna turned to me and said, *"I want the vacuum."*

It was the smoothest, easiest vacuum delivery imaginable. With a gentle pull, the baby emerged. He let out a cry, but it quickly faded. He went limp in my hands, his effortless delivery now a haunting contrast to his current condition.

I immediately began stimulating the baby, but he remained floppy, his tone nonexistent. The NICU team, already present, sprang into action. Our eyes met briefly as I clamped the cord, and Mark quickly cut it behind the clamp. The baby was handed off to the NICU team.

They worked tirelessly for 15 minutes, the longest minutes of my life. Then, finally, a muffled cry broke through the tension. Relief swept the room, but it was fleeting.

The baby was whisked to the NICU for cooling therapy. As I completed Johanna's perineal repair, anger welled within me. This was preventable. The vacuum had been so easy, so smooth—I could have delivered the baby over an hour earlier. The doula's insistence on *"no intervention"* had clouded the family's judgment, leading to unnecessary risk. It was a stark reminder that, while autonomy is crucial, it must be balanced with timely, informed decisions to ensure the safety of both mother and baby.

Reflection

Reflecting on the experience, I reaffirmed my commitment to setting clear boundaries and providing comprehensive education. Labor is unpredictable, and while most patients embrace a collaborative approach, rare cases like Johanna and Mark's underscore the importance of adaptability. My role is to guide families through turbulence, ensuring the safest landing for everyone on board.

The consequences were now stark. Unchecked misguided autonomy had jeopardized our sought outcome—a safe delivery for Johanna and her baby.

Chapter 10
The Breech Dilemma: A Story of Choice, Fear, and Triumph

Several times a month, I sit down with patients facing the unexpected reality of a breech presentation. I review the risks, the options, and—most importantly—the reality of what I can and cannot do; what I will and will not do. I always reassure them, *"I'm not a cowboy. A vaginal breech delivery only happens if it happens on its own."* Rules, precautions, and a deep commitment to safety guide every decision. In recent years, breech birth has gained attention, especially among Midwives. Yet, within hospitals and physician-led practices, resistance remains strong. Many providers refuse to attempt vaginal breech deliveries, leaving families with an impossible choice: accept a cesarean section or risk giving birth in a less structured, often unsafe environment. Some take that risk, and tragically, not all have happy endings.

Beatrice's Journey

Beatrice walked into my office at 35 weeks, desperate to avoid surgery. Her baby was breech. She had severe medical aversion—hospitals, needles, doctors—all of it terrified her. She had planned a home birth, but her Midwife, recognizing the limitations of out-of-hospital breech deliveries, sent her to me for a consultation.

Before meeting me, Beatrice had already spoken to another doctor. That conversation had left her discouraged. The doctor had told her to *"wait and see"* if the baby would turn, but dismissed the idea of an external cephalic version (ECV) to turn the baby manually. *"They don't work,"* he said. *"And you don't want me putting my body weight on your baby for 30 minutes trying to flip it."*

If she insisted, he'd do it—but only in the OR, under an epidural. Then came the discussion of breech delivery. His response was blunt: *"Absolutely not. No chance, no way."* A C-section was her only option unless nature intervened.

Beatrice and her partner sat before me, defeated but still hopeful. They needed an alternative.

A Different Conversation

Our discussion was long and thorough. I explained:

1. ACOG recommends offering ECV unless there is a valid contraindication.

2. When performed by a skilled provider, ECV is quick and does not require force. It is most successful around 36-37 weeks when fluid levels and fetal size are optimal.

3. I do not perform ECV in the OR under anesthesia unless specifically requested. I have seen too many *"Hollywood ECVs"* where the attempt is half-hearted, meant only to justify proceeding with the physician's preferred C-section.

4. If she chose to attempt a vaginal breech delivery, she needed to understand the risks. Head entrapment. Birth injuries. Even death.

I assured Beatrice I was not reckless—I follow strict criteria. But I also told her the truth: *"If you are admitted under my care, I will offer you a C-section first. The decision to proceed with vaginal breech delivery will be entirely yours."*

Despite the fear instilled by her previous doctor, Beatrice declined ECV. But she did feel safe enough to consider a vaginal breech birth.

The Birth

At 39 weeks and four days, Beatrice called me at 3 a.m. *"I think my water broke."*

She arrived at the hospital soaked in amniotic fluid—her membranes had ruptured. The baby was still breech. At her bedside, I made my standard offer: a primary C-section, the accepted norm in this community. I assured her that if she chose surgery, I would ensure it was as patient-centered.

Beatrice looked at me, calm and resolute. *"I understand the risks,"* she said. *"I want to try."*

She was 4cm dilated, laboring naturally. There was no augmentation—her body had to do this independently. She was offered an epidural for comfort and in case of an emergency, but she declined.

Less than six hours later, she was fully dilated and ready to push.

We moved to the OR—our safety net. The NICU team was on standby. My role was clear: I would guide Beatrice, but she had to be in control. Before any breech birth, I tell my patients:

"Know yourself. Know your pain tolerance. Know when you'll reach your limit—and be prepared to push 25% past it. If I tell you to turn, push, rotate, or stop, you must be able to do it. If at any point you can't, we move to a C-section. No questions, no hesitation. Safety first."

Beatrice understood. She was ready.

She pushed for just 15 minutes. And in those 15 minutes, she delivered her breech baby safely, without complication.

The Bigger Picture

Beatrice's story is not about defying medical norms. It is about informed choice. It is about creating space within the medical system for safe, evidence-based, and patient-centered options.

Not every breech baby should be born vaginally. Not every C-section is unnecessary. But when providers refuse to discuss options, when fear dictates decision-making, when families feel forced into surgery or out of the hospital altogether—that is when we fail.

Breech birth is not a reckless endeavor. It is a skill, a conversation, a collaboration.

And sometimes, when everything aligns—when patient, provider, and preparation come together—it is a triumph.

Informed Consent for Breech Vaginal Delivery and Breech Extraction

Your baby is in a breech presentation, meaning the baby's buttocks or feet are positioned to be delivered first instead of the head. The standard recommendation for breech presentation is cesarean delivery (C-section). However, in carefully selected patients, a vaginal breech delivery may be considered if certain conditions are met. This decision should be made based on risks, benefits, and your personal preferences in consultation with your Obstetric provider.

Current Standard of Care

The American College of Obstetricians and Gynecologists (ACOG) generally recommends C-section for breech presentation due to potential risks. However, ACOG supports attempts at vaginal breech delivery in tertiary care centers with experienced providers.

Important Considerations and Risks

If you choose to attempt a vaginal breech delivery, the following should be understood:

1. Medical Considerations and Risk Acknowledgment:

- Breech vaginal delivery is associated with potential complications, including:
    - Head entrapment, which may require emergency procedures that could affect future pregnancies.
    - Fractures (e.g., clavicle or humerus) or other birth injuries.
    - Cord prolapse, which can compromise the baby's oxygen supply and may require an emergency C-section.
    - Failure to progress or intolerance to labor, which may necessitate conversion to C-section.

- There are no options for labor induction or augmentation; spontaneous labor is required.
- Continuous fetal monitoring will assess the baby's well-being throughout labor.
- Delivery will occur in the operating room (OR) for immediate access to emergency C-section if needed.

2. Patient Selection and Requirements:

- **Motivated and Informed Patient:** Understanding the risks and being committed to the plan is essential.
- **Optimal Maternal Health:** No uncontrolled diabetes, excessive weight gain, or other conditions increasing risk.
- **Proven Pelvis:** A history of previous successful vaginal deliveries provides increased confidence in success.
- **Twin Considerations:** If delivering twins, a vaginal breech delivery is more favorable if both babies are of similar size **(concordant twins).**

3. Positioning of the Baby During Labor:

- The position of the baby will be evaluated throughout labor.

- If the baby transitions to an unstable or unfavorable position, an immediate C-section may be recommended.

4. Situations Requiring Immediate Cesarean Section:

- Footling or double footling breech presentation (risk of cord prolapse and delivery complications).- *Though with more detailed and thoughtful counselling this also remains an option in some instances.*
- Transverse lie (baby is positioned sideways, making vaginal delivery impossible).
- Non-reassuring fetal heart tones (suggesting the baby is distressed and requires immediate intervention).
- Failure to progress, dilate, or prolonged labor (increasing risk of complications).
- Umbilical cord prolapse (cutting off oxygen supply to the baby).

Patient Acknowledgment and Consent

I have been counseled on the risks, benefits, and alternatives to breech vaginal delivery, including the option for a planned cesarean section. I understand that:

- A C-section remains the community standard of care for breech presentation.
- Vaginal breech delivery carries increased risks compared to head-first (cephalic) vaginal delivery.
- I may require an emergency C-section if complications arise.
- My provider will make real-time decisions to ensure the safety of both me and my baby.

I have had the opportunity to ask questions and understand the information presented. I voluntarily agree to proceed with a trial of vaginal breech delivery under the conditions outlined above.

Informed Consent for Trial of Labor After Cesarean (TOLAC)

You have a history of a prior cesarean section and are considering a Trial of Labor After Cesarean (TOLAC) to achieve a vaginal birth after cesarean (VBAC). The success rate for VBAC is approximately 80%, with a 20% failure rate, including 15% for non-emergent indications (e.g., failure to progress) and less than 2% for emergent situations (e.g., placental abruption, uterine rupture). My role is to provide you with a clear understanding of the risks and benefits so that you can make an informed decision that aligns with the safety and well-being of both you and your baby.

Our Approach to Care

1. I have explained in detail that I cannot predict whether you will have a successful VBAC or require a repeat C-section.

2. I have outlined my approach to labor management:

   - I will attempt to be in-house by 6cm dilation or active labor if it is progressing rapidly.

   - Continuous fetal monitoring is essential to detect signs of distress or complications.

   - TOLAC will occur at a tertiary care center where immediate surgical intervention is available.

3. My role is to provide an accurate risk-benefit analysis for every decision made during labor. You can decide the best course for you and your family, provided the decision-making is based on safety and informed choice.

Risks, Benefits, and Alternatives Informed (RBAI) Discussion

TOLAC or VBAC Risks and Benefits:

☑ **Benefits:**

- 80% success rate.

- Faster recovery compared to C-section.
- Reduced maternal morbidity (lower risk of infection, hemorrhage, and complications in future pregnancies).
- Lower risk of surgical complications.

⚠ **Risks:**

- 20% failure rate, with 15% due to non-emergent reasons and 5% requiring emergency intervention.
- Risk of uterine rupture (0.5-1%), which may require emergency C-section and can lead to serious maternal or fetal complications.
- Increased risk of fetal distress requiring urgent intervention.
- Labor dystocia or failed progression, necessitating repeat C-section.

Planned Repeat C-section Risks and Benefits:

✅ **Benefits:**

- Planned procedure with a controlled surgical environment.
- Avoidance of labor-related complications.

- Elimination of uterine rupture risk.

⚠ **Risks:**

- Increased risk of surgical complications (infection, hemorrhage, adhesions).
- Longer recovery time compared to vaginal birth.
- Potential complications in future pregnancies (placenta accreta, increased risk of hysterectomy).

Ongoing Prenatal Care and Preparation

1. Pregnancy Beyond 36 Weeks: Maternal and fetal risks increase with prolonged pregnancy. While there is no immediate need for induction in many cases, we encourage natural preparation for labor (e.g., regular intercourse) to help prevent late-term deliveries and associated complications. Goal delivery 38-39 weeks in natural labor

Patient Acknowledgment and Consent

I have been counseled on the risks, benefits, and alternatives of TOLAC versus elective repeat cesarean delivery. I understand that:

- VBAC has an 80% success rate, but failure may result in repeat C-section, including emergency surgery.

- Uterine rupture, while rare, is a serious risk requiring immediate intervention.
- I will be closely monitored, and safety is the priority in all decisions made during labor.
- My provider will remain available and present during active labor to ensure prompt care.

I have had the opportunity to ask questions and understand the information presented. I voluntarily agree to proceed with a trial of labor after cesarean (TOLAC) under the conditions outlined above.

The balance between patient choice, medical expertise, and the risks involved in breech deliveries. It emphasizes the importance of informed consent, open communication, and patient-centered care, where the provider guides but ultimately respects the patient's decision. The cases discussed demonstrate the significance of experience and the need for careful consideration when deciding breach presentations, especially in a hospital setting. The story of April's VBAC delivery and Beatrice's Breech delivery are testaments to how, when safety measures are in place, trusting the patient's wishes and empowering them with knowledge can lead to successful outcomes, challenging the traditional norms and offering an alternative to standard practices.

Chapter 11
The Importance of Detailed Conversations and the Soft-Landing Approach

In my practice, detailed discussions about birth plans are not just routine—they are essential. These conversations allow time for all participants to ask questions, align their expectations, and, most importantly, ensure that both parents are on the same page. Often, mothers and fathers enter these discussions with vastly different understandings, emotions, and concerns.

My consents serve as more than just legal documentation—they provide a *"soft landing"* for those who choose a path outside the traditional standard of care. They offer a balance: access to safe, skilled medical care while honoring a patient's autonomy. This approach allows for individualized care plans, even when they diverge from the rigid guidelines of ACOG.

In my experience, most patients who initially want something outside of standard practice often change course when labor truly begins. The pain, intensity, and unpredictability—many quickly opt for more conventional options. But for the small percentage who persist and hold firm in their choices, they tend to do well. Their motivation and stamina carry them through.

However, the ones who concern me most are those whose determination crosses into rigidity—those who refuse to yield to nature's course, resisting even in the face of medical urgency. The emotional toll of an unfulfilled birth plan can be devastating. I have heard women, tears streaming down their faces, whisper, *"I am a failure,"* or, *"I am not a real woman."* The belief that vaginal birth, unmedicated birth, is a badge of honor weighs heavily. And when that perceived badge is not earned, it can break them.

Our tertiary care center should serve as a refuge, offering safety, expertise, and compassion. Our team is committed to creating a judgment-free space where every woman feels seen and heard. Many of our patients come with unique histories—deep-seated traumas, cultural influences, or prior negative medical experiences. Some struggle with reconciling their ideal birth experience with the realities of medical necessity. We aim to meet them where they are, blending evidence-based care with genuine respect for personal autonomy.

One way to ensure this "soft landing" is through co-management—a model that fosters trust between patients and providers long before labor begins. When a patient enters birth with an established relationship with her provider and care team, safety is no longer just a checklist—it becomes an integrated, living part of the plan.

It's much like teaching a child to ride a bike. You don't wait until they're speeding downhill to start giving instructions. You begin on flat ground, hand on the seat, offering steady guidance. At first, they may wobble or fall, but your presence gives them confidence. They trust you to catch them, correct them, and encourage them. And slowly, they begin to pedal forward on their own.

In the same way, patients need to feel their providers steady presence from the beginning—before the chaos, the complications, and the critical choices. Trust built early allows patients to lean in when it matters most. And just like the hand on the bike seat, that trust doesn't control—it supports, guides, and eventually lets go at the right moment, when the rider is ready to move forward with confidence and autonomy.

Stephanie's Story

Stephanie came to me seeking co-management. She wanted a home birth, but she was also high-risk.

This was her sixth pregnancy. Her first birth had been traumatic—a cesarean was performed under rushed circumstances due to non-reassuring fetal heart tones. She had received an epidural, and the baby's heart rate plummeted to the 50s and never recovered. She was rushed into surgery, where they performed a T-incision on her uterus. Afterward, she was told she could never attempt a vaginal birth again.

Her second pregnancy resulted in another C-section—her provider refused to entertain the idea of a VBAC.

By her third pregnancy, Stephanie had lost all trust in the medical system. She delivered alone at home (Free Birth). Both she and the baby did well.

For her fourth and fifth pregnancies, she sought the care of a Midwife but still refused hospital intervention. Her Catholic faith prevented her from using contraception, and now, at an advanced maternal age, she found herself pregnant again, with a history of three successful VBACs on a T-incision uterus.

At 32 weeks, her baby was breech. With reluctance, her Midwife advised her to establish co-care with me.

Each time she sat in my office, she made it clear: *"I don't need you. I can do this. I know my body."*

At 39 weeks and five days, she was sent to me by her Midwife with severe blood pressure. An ultrasound confirmed that her baby had turned cephalic. Yet Stephanie was in denial. She believed she would be forced into a C-section.

I offered hospitalization for close monitoring. She refused. She left against medical advice.

Two days later, she returned to OB triage with a severe headache. Her blood pressure was dangerously high, and her liver enzymes were elevated. She had severe preeclampsia. She needed to deliver.

For any patient with a T-incision uterus, standard care dictates a C-section to avoid uterine rupture. But Stephanie had successfully delivered vaginally three times before. She refused surgery.

I could not, in good conscience, induce or augment her labor—if she ruptured, I would have contributed to that outcome. Yet she refused intervention.

The tension in the room was palpable. The nurses were visibly uneasy. My team was on edge. Maternal-Fetal Medicine was called to the bedside.

For four hours, we debated, discussed, and stalled. Meanwhile, her cervix had progressed from 3cm to 6cm despite contractions being infrequent.

I made the call. I moved her to a labor room.

I offered artificial rupture of membranes—a controlled step that could allow her body to progress naturally. She agreed.

Within one hour, she delivered vaginally—uncomplicated.

Reflection and Lessons from Stephanie

I often remind my residents that preeclampsia does not mean a C-section. It means delivery.

The body often knows it is sick and will work to relieve itself of the illness. Our job, sometimes, is to get out of the way.

I also remind my patients that when I say *"induction of labor,"* I don't always mean medication or intervention. Sometimes, it simply means going to the hospital, where we can monitor, assess, and act quickly if needed. It means being in a safe place, whether or not they choose to accept the care we offer.

For Stephanie, her trauma was so pervasive, so deeply ingrained, that safety could only be achieved through an alternative plan—one that honored her autonomy while still ensuring the best possible outcome, individualized care.

In the end, safety and autonomy are not mutually exclusive. The best care is the one that allows both to coexist.

Chapter 12

Life and Death: Real Conversations in Maternal Care

In life and death moments, that's when the real challenges of the right of patients to decide for themselves hit the hardest.

I remember Mavis. She came into the hospital quietly, almost casually, complaining of decreased fetal movement. This was her third pregnancy. She wasn't new to the game — she knew how babies moved, how their tone and energy shifted. She had an anterior placenta, which I had explained could sometimes soften the way movements felt, almost muffling the baby's kicks. Still, what she was describing was different.

The baby was 34 weeks. For three days, Mavis said, she hadn't felt the usual strong surges or fluttery shifts. She thought maybe it was normal. Perhaps the appointment she had scheduled for the next day would clear things up. But something — perhaps instinct — had nudged her in earlier.

We put her on the monitor immediately. The NST was non-reactive, and the strip was almost a flat line. A biophysical profile (BPP) was ordered stat. The score came back: 2 out of 8. Not good.

They called me to the bedside urgently. I moved quickly, knowing we were losing precious time.

Standing next to Mavis, I explained, as calmly and clearly as I could, that we needed to deliver her baby by emergency C-section. Mavis hesitated. She had delivered naturally before, had always trusted her body, and now struggled to see the emergency in a moment that still felt so still, so unreal.

I broke it down for her.

"Do you know what a BPP is really asking?" I asked gently.

She hesitated, unsure.

"It's asking: Is the baby sick?" I continued.

Still unsure, she looked at me. So I tried again.

"When you're sick, what do you do?"

She paused, thinking. "I guess... I stay in bed. Try to sleep it off."

"Exactly," I said. "When we're sick, our bodies slow down to conserve energy. We move less. We eat and drink less. We rest. Babies do the same. When they're unwell, they stop practicing breathing. They stop moving. Their tone decreases. The fluid around them drops. These are the signs we measure during a Biophysical Profile — or BPP. We look at breathing, movement, tone, and amniotic fluid. Each is a signal."

I watched her absorb it, then explained further. "A perfect score is 8 out of 8. That tells us the baby is well, usually for at least 72 hours. A score of 6 means we need to monitor closely. Four or lower usually means the baby is in distress, and we need to deliver."

She grew quiet. A long, heavy pause filled the room as she weighed the information.

Then she nodded.

We rushed to the OR.

Her baby was delivered limp, silent. No cry. The NICU team stepped in immediately, resuscitating and stabilizing the baby. Mavis cried — deep, shaking sobs — not just from fear, but from overwhelming gratitude. Gratitude that she had come in that night instead of waiting until morning.

That moment stayed with me. It changed how I practiced.

After that, I made a promise: every patient would understand fetal movement and the meaning of a BPP long before they ever faced an emergency.

So we built it into our care.

I started teaching the signs in the clinic:

- After 20 weeks, you'll feel flutters.
- Each week, those movements grow stronger and more regular.
- By 30 weeks, movement should be constant—rolling, kicking, stretching.
- Babies do sleep—but in short cycles, usually 20–40 minutes. Outside of that, you should feel movement.
- It's not about how *strong* the kicks feel. It's about how *consistent* they are.

If a baby's pattern changes — if the rhythm the mother knows so well suddenly slows or stops — that's not something to wait on. That's the alarm bell.

Judy learned that lesson well.

She had received the same education during her prenatal visits. One evening, she noticed her baby wasn't moving like usual. It had only been four hours, but something felt off.

Judy didn't wait.

She came straight to the hospital.

This was her second pregnancy, and she had an anterior placenta — something that already made feeling movement a little harder. But she knew what her baby's patterns normally felt like. Despite all the usual tricks — juice, cold water, lying on her side — the baby stayed quiet that night.

I ordered an urgent BPP. The results came back: 4 out of 8. She was only 32 weeks. This baby was in trouble.

We moved quickly—emergency C-section.

When I delivered the baby, I found the umbilical cord wrapped tightly around the baby's neck five times.

Five.

The NICU team was ready. Despite being premature, this baby fought hard. After weeks of care and monitoring, that baby went home — healthy, thriving, a fighter.

Every year since, I get a Christmas card from Judy. And every year, a smiling face looks back at me — a reminder of the power of education, instinct, and trust.

That baby survived because Judy listened to her gut — and because we had built the kind of relationship where she *knew* it was okay to come in. She knew her concern would be taken seriously.

Stories like these aren't just about emergency saves. They're about what's possible when patients are informed and empowered — and when providers truly listen.

Not every story ends with a happy ending..

Recently, a new challenge emerged that tested the limits of patient autonomy and provider responsibility.

A patient arrived at the hospital already in active labor. She had planned a home birth, fully aware that her baby was breech. She'd undergone two external cephalic versions (ECVs) in the weeks prior, both unsuccessful. Still, she remained resolute in her decision to attempt a vaginal delivery.

When I met her at the bedside, she was nearly ready to push. I reviewed her options again, calmly but thoroughly. I offered a C-section, explaining the risks of a vaginal breech birth: the potential for cord prolapse, head entrapment, and traumatic injury. She nodded—she had heard all of this before—and signed an Against Medical Advice (AMA) form, reaffirming her decision to proceed with a vaginal birth.

Labor progressed quickly. But as she began to push, fatigue crept in. Her confidence wavered.

"I can't," she whispered, defeated. "I can't do this."

At that moment, there was no space for confusion or pause.

"If you feel you cannot continue," I told her gently but firmly, "then we have to move to an emergency C-section now. This moment is not safe for you or your baby. We can't linger in indecision."

Something shifted in her eyes. A spark of clarity. She gathered her strength.

With fierce determination, she pushed with everything she had. And moments later, she delivered her breech baby vaginally—beautifully, safely, without complication.

The line between triumph and tragedy had been razor-thin. But she crossed it with full autonomy, informed strength, and unwavering support at her side.

Later that night, I was called back for another patient. Diane.

She was 31 weeks pregnant and had been feeling decreased fetal movement for over two days. She hadn't come in sooner, hoping things would return to normal. But now, she was worried.

The non-stress test (NST) showed a Category III tracing—ominous and urgent. Her biophysical profile was 4 out of 8. These were warning signs we could not ignore.

I sat beside her and spoke with honesty and compassion.

"There are two kinds of families in moments like these," I said softly. "One acts immediately, knowing that each minute matters. The other waits—hoping for more clarity, more reassurance—while precious time slips away."

She listened quietly, the weight of the moment sinking in.

After a long breath, Diane made her decision.

We moved swiftly to the operating room. Her baby was delivered by C-section—silent, limp, but with a heartbeat.

The NICU team took over instantly. Intubation. Oxygen. Every effort to coax life back into that fragile body.

And slowly, the baby responded.

That child survived not because we had all the answers, but because Diane made a choice when it mattered most. Because we moved.

Two stories. One theme.

In one case, a mother insisted on a path most would reject—and she triumphed.

In the other, a mother surrendered to the urgency of the unknown—and saved her child.

Both trusted themselves. Both were fully supported by a team that respected their autonomy and strength.

And both remind us that maternal care is never one-size-fits-all. It is a careful dance of knowledge, trust, courage, and timing, where decisions shape outcomes and how those decisions are made and honored.

Life Lessons that shape my practice:

Lesson 1

Years ago, when I was still a young doctor, I learned a lesson that has stayed with me ever since—one that changed the way I speak to patients forever.

I was on the medicine floor, presenting a case to my senior resident. The patient was a man with end-stage liver failure. He drank heavily and was frequently in and out of the hospital. I gave the full report—labs, vitals, imaging, medications—but then my resident asked a question that caught me completely off guard:

"Did you tell him he could die?"

I paused. The air felt heavy. I hadn't said those words. I had talked about risks, about prognosis, about organ function—but not death.

I was scared. Scared to say it out loud. Scared of what it might mean for him. For me. For both of us.

But my resident didn't let it go. He looked me straight in the eye and said, firmly:

"Sometimes you have to say the word: death. Patients deserve the truth—even when it's hard. Especially when it's hard."

That moment never left me.

Years later, I find myself facing the same dilemma—but now, it's often with pregnant patients, expectant mothers, families on the edge of hope and fear. And somehow, the conversation feels even heavier.

Telling a mother that her baby could die feels like violating something sacred. It feels too raw, too harsh—like you're puncturing a fragile bubble of hope. I even wonder if I am propagating fear tactics.

It's easier to soften the language. To say "concern," or "complication," or "monitoring." It's tempting to wrap the truth in gentle phrases, to circle around it rather than land directly on it.

But if we only whisper around the truth—if we're vague or evasive in our language—we leave families in a fog of uncertainty. We confuse them. We strip them of the chance to understand the gravity of the moment and make fully informed decisions. And we risk losing time—time that, in many cases, we can't afford to lose.

The truth is: our job isn't just to heal. It's to speak clearly in moments that matter most.

Not to scare, but to prepare.

Not to pressure, but to empower.

Not to take hope away, but to make room for courage—real courage, rooted in truth.

That lesson—learned in a crowded hospital hallway from a mentor who wasn't afraid to speak plainly—guides me still. It reminds me that compassion is not the absence of truth. It is the delivery of truth with clarity, kindness, and the respect every patient deserves.

Lesson 2

Growing up, I learned something else about communication—something that didn't come from textbooks or classrooms, but from my own family.

My brother and I were close, but we were different in almost every way. He was the athlete—charismatic, physical, instinctive. I was the dreamer and the academic, always chasing ideas and books.

One year after struggling through a rigorous private school curriculum, my brother was given a second chance: he could finish at a public school with a lighter course load. It was an opportunity to reset—to succeed on his own terms.

But he blew it.

I came home from college and heard he was failing again. I was furious. Disappointed. Heartbroken.

We were driving to Blockbuster—yes, it was that long ago—and I just erupted. I yelled at him, screamed at the steering wheel, and pounded it in frustration. I was overwhelmed by what felt like wasted potential, a door closing that he might never get back.

When we got home, he casually walked into the house, frustrated, and said to my mom, "Michael's going crazy!"

That was the moment I realized something painful and important:

He hadn't heard my concern.
He hadn't felt my love.
He only heard my anger.

All the things I meant to say—the frustration rooted in love, the urgency born from belief in him—got lost in the delivery.

In maternal care, it's exactly the same.

It's not enough to know the science or to understand the risk.
It's not enough to care deeply.

If we don't communicate in a way that families can receive, they won't hear our wisdom or concern—they'll only hear judgment, fear, or shame.

Our words must carry both weight and warmth, especially in moments where life and death hang in the balance.

It's not just about delivering the truth.
It's about delivering it in a way they can *hear*.
In a way that allows them to *understand.*
In a way that empowers them to *act*—without shutting down, without turning away.

That lesson, first taught to me in the front seat of a car on a random night, echoes every time I walk into a room holding hard news. Because in medicine—as in life—how we speak matters as much as *what* we say.

Conclusion

Conclusion: Speaking Truth with Compassion

The stories above, from medical emergencies to personal memories, all point to one essential truth: *how* we communicate is just as important as *what* we communicate, especially in moments of crisis.

Whether we are telling a mother that her baby may not survive or urging a family to make an urgent decision, our delivery determines whether that truth will be heard, trusted, and acted upon. Fear and urgency must never overshadow empathy and respect. If they do, the message will be lost.

Families don't respond to clinical jargon or blunt warnings. They respond to clarity, honesty, and compassion. They need to feel our concern, not just hear our expertise.

We hold powerful knowledge as providers, but it's meaningless if we can't translate it into a human connection. This is the heart of maternal care: not just guiding patients through birth, but standing beside them, speaking hard truths in soft ways, and helping them feel seen, heard, and empowered to choose the path that's right for them.

Because in the end, it's not just about saving lives—it's about honoring the ones who live them.

Chapter 13

Strange Autonomy

It's always a challenge when new patients come to my practice after transferring care from another provider, often for the simple yet profound reason that they didn't feel heard. Time and time again, I hear patients say they brought in a birth plan, asked about labor options like movement, intermittent monitoring, or birthing positions, and were met with resistance, dismissal, or outright denial. Many describe rigid environments where control seems to outweigh compassion.

One story still rings in my ears: a Spanish-speaking mother in labor, visited by a physician who didn't speak her language. He requested an amniotomy, reached for the hook, and when she voiced her refusal — clearly and repeatedly — the nurse translated her words, "No, I don't want that." The physician disregarded her autonomy, responded coldly, "She doesn't get to decide. I'm the doctor," and ruptured her membranes anyway.

These are real stories. And they are devastating.

Empathy and compassion are not optional in our field. They are necessary. Allowing a person to walk into your care environment

— vulnerable, hopeful, afraid — and honoring their goals, preferences, and sense of self is humbling. Sometimes, it is even uncomfortable. But always necessary.

I remember a woman who came to my clinic hoping for a natural, undisturbed birth. It was her second pregnancy. Unwanted interventions had marred her first, and now she simply wanted to be left alone. Her birth plan was short and simple: "Please don't bother me unless medically necessary."

She arrived at the hospital in the middle of the night, wearing a pink and grey Ralph Lauren sweatsuit, sunglasses, hoodie up, her hair pulled back. She grunted with each contraction, declined a cervical check, and refused an IV. She lay on the triage bed, legs crossed, hood up, sweatpants and shoes still on — silent except for her primal vocalizations.

The staff was unsure what to do. I reviewed her birth plan, introduced myself gently, and asked how she was doing. "Fine," she said. "I just want to be left alone."

Her husband stood at her side, rubbing her back through each contraction. Time passed. Without fanfare, she pulled off her sweatpants, lowered herself to the floor, and delivered her baby with grace and quiet power. Afterward, she looked up at us and said, "That was the best delivery I've ever had. Exactly what I wanted." She plans to return for every future birth.

And then there's the Swiss couple — another story of what I now call "strange autonomy." They came to the U.S. from a country where birth is predominantly Midwife-led, hands-off, and respectful of the natural process. They'd seen multiple doctors in Phoenix and finally landed in our practice after hearing that we do things a bit differently.

When labor began, she came to the hospital already completely dilated — and brought with her a doula who looked like she'd stepped straight out of a BBC period film: hair in a tight bun, soft-spoken, hands folded in her lap. Her demeanor was calm but firm. The patient sat in the wheelchair and refused to move to the bed.

At first, I thought, "This will be a beautiful birth — she labored at home, arrived complete, all we have to do is catch." But hours passed. She wouldn't move. She said she physically couldn't. An hour became two, then four. Meanwhile, I delivered two other patients. She remained in the chair, quiet, alert, but unmoving.

I tried humor — "It's hard to deliver a baby from a rolling chair" — and even she chuckled. Still, she wasn't ready. I gave her more time. After six hours had passed, she finally moved to bed. But despite full dilation, she didn't push. She didn't want coaching. No directed pushing. No counting. No pressure. Just time.

I tried again: "May I help you?" They listened. Finally, she agreed to let me guide her with some gentle counterpressure and coaching.

Fifteen minutes later, she delivered. She and her husband were overjoyed. They thanked me not just for the safe outcome but also for the space, the patience, and the willingness to try it their way first.

She later developed pelvic pain and required physical therapy — a reminder that autonomy doesn't mean perfect outcomes. But the gratitude remained. She felt heard. She felt supported. She felt respected.

Conclusion

Strange autonomy is not really so strange at all. It's simply what happens when patients refuse to surrender their humanity to systems that too often forget it. These stories remind me that the role of a provider isn't just to deliver babies — it's to deliver care that honors a person's right to choose how they move through one of the most intimate, vulnerable, and powerful moments of their life.

Autonomy doesn't mean chaos. It doesn't mean rejecting medical advice or abandoning safety. It means walking with someone, not over them. And when we choose to respect that — even when it challenges us — we create not just better outcomes, but better memories, better trust, and a better kind of medicine.

Chapter 14

Gentle C-Section: A Misnomer with Real Meaning

I've shared the story of how I entered Obstetrics and Gynecology many times. When I first entered medical school, I was convinced I would become an oncologist—more specifically, a radiation oncologist. I fell in love with the field while working with some of the most phenomenal physicians in Atlanta, Georgia—Dr. Jerome Landry, Dr. Tucker, Dr. Holmes, and many others. They practiced with such intellect and compassion that I saw a future there for myself, filled with research, patient advocacy, and meaningful care.

So when we were instructed to choose our least likely specialty as our first clinical rotation, the idea was to develop the necessary rounding, presenting, and shadowing skills early—skills that would help us thrive once we reached our intended field. I chose OB/GYN without hesitation. There was *no way* I was going to be dealing with pregnant women, navigating their very personal experiences, or managing their deliveries. OB/GYN, I thought, was just not for me.

But then came my third day. I was assigned to the surgical suite and given the opportunity to observe my first cesarean section. Up to that point, I'd never been in an operating room. I had imagined surgery to be pristine, delicate, and meticulous. Instead, I saw two very petite women—an attending and a resident—stand on either side of a laboring mother. They cut, stretched, pulled, and worked in unison to deliver a baby. They worked quickly, efficiently, and with confidence. Then they replaced, sutured, trimmed, and restored the anatomy with a rhythm that was almost musical. They explained each step to me as they worked.

I walked out of that room completely in awe.

That night, I called my father, excited, passionate, and full of conviction. I had witnessed something transformative—something messy, powerful, and deeply human. From that moment on, I knew I wanted to be an OB/GYN. I spent the rest of that rotation ducking sniper threats between West Virginia and Maryland (yes, *that* infamous 2002 sniper episode), just to get to the hospital and be part of the next delivery.

So when a family comes to me now—whether they've had three prior C-sections or are facing a new set of risks or realities—I often hear them say they want something different this time. Many ask for a "gentle C-section." And I'll be honest: I often push back on that term.

There is no such thing, technically, as a *gentle* C-section. But there *is* such a thing as a **patient-centered** one.

Every surgery is surgery. The scalpel is sharp. The technique is precise. The risks are real. But the experience that can be shaped.

When I hear a family request a gentle C-section, I don't dismiss it. Instead, I dig deeper: *What is it you're really asking for? What would make this feel more like your birth, your moment, your story?*

From there, I offer a list of elements that can enhance the experience:

- **Lighting**: We dim the overhead lights and only illuminate the surgical field. It removes the harsh glare and sterile feel, making the room feel less like an interrogation chamber and more like a safe space.

- **Music**: Whether it's gospel, jazz, or a favorite pop song, curated music transforms the tone of the room. For some, its a spiritual balm. For others, it 's a calming anchor.

- **Delayed Cord Clamping**: Even in surgery, I strive to allow the cord to stay intact until it turns white. I educate families: 500 mL of blood flows to the uterus per minute. Letting the baby receive even just 90 seconds of delayed clamping provides significant benefits.

- **Cord Cutting**: Sometimes, we leave the cord long enough for mom or a partner to participate in trimming it, adding another point of connection to the experience.

- **Skin-to-Skin**: My personal goal is five minutes. After vitals and basic assessments, the baby should be on the mother's chest. Even in the OR, this kind of bonding is achievable.

- **Assisted Delivery (Under Development)**: Our hospital is working on protocols allowing mothers to assist in their delivery. Through a sterile drape with a built-in panel, the mother can reach down and bring her baby to her chest, reclaiming a piece of what's often lost in the operating room.

These steps don't erase the surgical nature of a C-section. They don't make it "gentle" in the literal sense. However, they do center the patient and family in the experience. They turn a procedure into a memory shaped by warmth, agency, and compassion.

Conclusion: Honoring the Humanity in Surgery

A C-section is still a C-section. The incision is still made. The uterus still bleeds. The surgeon still pulls and tucks, replaces and sutures. But when we listen and take the time to understand what a family needs to feel connected to their birth, we create something more than a routine operation. We create an experience that honors the humanity of everyone involved.

That's what I strive for—not a gentle C-section, but a *purposeful* one. A *patient-centered* one. And perhaps, in that deeper intention, we find a gentleness that surgery alone could never provide.

Chapter 15

Difficult Stories in Autonym: How I Navigate.

A Birth on the Brink

Lisa arrived at the hospital in tears. At 42 weeks and three days into her first pregnancy, she had envisioned a peaceful home birth, surrounded by familiar faces and the care of her chosen Midwife. Her pregnancy had been smooth, at least on the surface. But as I looked through her records, gaps in her prenatal care stood out: no diabetes screening, no Group B strep test, only a single hemoglobin check at the start of her pregnancy. Still, she had trusted the plan. She had done everything she was supposed to.

Now, she was here, frustrated and heartbroken. At 42 weeks, her dream of delivering at home was no longer viable. She had heard about me—how I supported natural birth within the hospital—and she clung to the hope that showing up at our clinic would mean finding the right team to guide her through.

I sat beside her as she wiped away her tears. My first words to her were crucial but straightforward: *"This is a safe place."* I wanted her to know that her goals mattered and that her birth plan would be honored as much as possible. That she and her baby would be safe. Her body. Her choice. My job was not to dictate but to educate—to help her make informed decisions, never to force a course of action she didn't want.

Relief softened her face. Slowly, the tension in the room eased. Lisa's husband, a quiet but steady presence, nodded in agreement as they handed me their birth plan. It outlined their wishes: no Pitocin, no unnecessary interventions, the list of "nos" was innumerable. I carefully reviewed it, pausing midway.

"Tell me about the yeses," I said.

Lisa's eyes widened, then softened. She and her husband spoke about movement, showering during labor, and their doula's presence. They wanted an active, hands-on experience. I listened, then gently explained the reality of where we stood. At 42 weeks, certain risks loomed—low fluid, an aging placenta, and a baby that might not tolerate labor well. I assured them that we would work together, balancing their wishes with what was safest.

We discussed induction methods. I explained the options, their benefits, and their drawbacks. Cytotec was effective but irreversible once given. The Cervidil tampon could be removed, but its effects would linger, like a burning ember, even after being taken out. Pitocin, however, gave us control. We could start, stop, or adjust. Most mothers did well with it, though a small percentage didn't. I promised them they would have control. No one would force anything on them.

Hours later, Lisa and her husband made their decision—Pitocin. When I checked on them, she was progressing. A few hours in, her water broke. The fluid was scant, but the baby looked stable. She requested that the Pitocin be turned off. No one questioned it; her wishes were respected.

Three hours later, the call came: she was fully dilated and feeling pushy. When I entered the room, Lisa knelt over a squat bar, her husband in front of her, forehead to forehead, whispering encouragement. She bore down, grunting with each contraction. The room was quiet except for her labors rhythmic rise and fall .

At first, progress was steady. Then it stalled. Ten minutes passed. Then another ten. The baby wasn't moving down.

"This is the hardest part," I told her. *"You have to push through this. I know it hurts, but this is when it counts the most."*

She listened. With the next contraction, she pushed with everything she had. The baby's body was delivered with ease, slipping onto the bed between her knees. Lisa rocked back on her heels, reaching for her child, bringing the baby to her chest as we stimulated for a cry.

Nothing.

The room fell silent.

The little body was limp, eyes open but unseeing.

"We need to move—now."

Cord clamped. Cut. Baby rushed to the warmer. The NICU team arrived within seconds. One minute passed. Two. The heartbeat was strong, but the baby was unresponsive. No breathing. No tone. The same quiet stillness we had seen on the monitor.

They suctioned once, twice, retrieving a rush of fluid. A gasp. A soft cry. Another puff of CPAP, and color returned. Dusky purple turned to pink.

A collective exhale filled the room. Relief washed over everyone—Lisa, her husband, the nurses, the Midwife, and me. Had this happened at home, the outcome could have been drastically different.

That night, the medical team urged further monitoring. Shock at birth warranted caution, even if the baby now appeared well. But to our surprise, Lisa and her husband declined. The next day, as I rounded, I learned they had chosen to leave against medical advice. They refused further testing despite the blood gas results being concerning.

I discharged Lisa—there was no medical reason to keep her. The baby was beyond my jurisdiction. At the very least, I urged them to stay one more night. But their minds were made up.

Before they left, Lisa and her husband thanked me. They expressed gratitude for the care they had received. They were thankful they had been in the hospital, yet they still believed their baby was fine. I didn't push. I didn't argue. I provided information, respected their autonomy, and let them go.

But I couldn't shake the thought—would this story have ended the same way if they had been at home?

A Birth Against the Odds

Jared and his wife met me in the clinic approximately 26 weeks into their pregnancy. Jared was a highly educated physics professor at the local university, deeply respected both professionally and within his church community. His young bride of less than a year found herself unexpectedly pregnant, and together, they were elated at the opportunity to grow their family. Naturally minded, they had set their hearts on a home birth.

There was just one problem—Jared and his wife were expecting natural triplets.

Initially, they sought care from a highly respected Midwife in the community. She had agreed to monitor the pregnancy for the first few months, understanding that things could change quickly. By the later part of the second trimester, she strongly urged them to transition their care to my team.

When they arrived at my office, they were excited yet cautious. Jared, protective of his wife, carried a quiet but firm presence. I approached them with respect and education, as I did all my patients, never coercion.

"I'm not here to tell you what to do," I assured them. *"My goal is to provide you with options—safe mom, safe babies. You have choices."*

They immediately laid out their expectations. *"Under absolutely no circumstances do we want a C-section,"* Jared insisted. *"We want labor to begin naturally. No unnecessary interventions."*

We discussed their birth plan in detail—delayed cord clamping, immediate skin-to-skin, and minimal medical interference. The one medical concern hovering over the pregnancy was Jared's wife's narcolepsy. She was on several stimulants and neuro medications, but after discussion, we believed the risks to be manageable.

They acclimated well to our clinic, attending routine evaluations and seeing a high-risk specialist for monitoring. The Maternal-Fetal Medicine team confirmed that all three babies had their own placentas—a favorable scenario. Their recommendation was clear: delivery should occur around 36 to 37 weeks via c-section.

Jared was immediately resistant. *"We trust you,"* he said, *"But we don't want to be rushed into anything."*

I reassured them that we would handle their care thoughtfully. They requested their Midwife be present at delivery, which we accommodated. The pregnancy remained uncomplicated until 36 weeks and five days, when she arrived in active labor.

A Room Packed with Anticipation

Labor progressed naturally, and she adamantly refused any augmentation. The OR was prepped for delivery—standing room only. Three separate fetal monitors tracked the babies' heartbeats. A complete medical team stood by, ready for any complication: surgical scrubs for a potential emergency C-section, an anesthesiologist, and a CRNA on standby, neonatal teams prepared for three premature newborns, multiple OB-GYNs, me, and a fleet of nurses. The atmosphere was thick with anticipation.

She pushed for about 30 to 45 minutes before Baby A arrived, head down, crying, and with a long, healthy cord. I placed the baby on her chest.

Then came Baby B.

I offered an intervention, but I wasn't sure she fully grasped the moment—she was unmedicated, had no epidural, and was lost in the intensity of labor. I reached inside, ruptured the sac, and guided Baby B, who was breech. The baby was born safely and placed on her chest. Meanwhile, Baby A was taken to the warmer for evaluation.

Now, Baby C.

I asked for permission to proceed. She hesitated but nodded. I broke the amniotic sac and found Baby C positioned high. I had her push while I maneuvered the baby downward. Fifteen minutes passed. Baby B was moved from her chest to be evaluated at that time. Jared was running between his wife and the two babies, his excitement evident, but his anxiety growing.

Then, suddenly, Baby C's heart tones dropped—and they didn't recover.

My mind raced. Once stretched to capacity, the uterus rapidly contracted around three separate placentas. The risk of placental abruption was very real.

"I need a vacuum," I called.

Within seconds, it was in my hands. I applied it to Baby C's head and, with controlled force, guided the baby out. A moment of silence—and then a strong cry. Baby C was placed on his mother's chest, the umbilical cord still attached. Relief flooded the room.

Jared's face, however, was tense. Anger flickered in his eyes.

"This wasn't what we wanted," he said, voice tight with frustration.

I met his gaze, steady but firm. *"In an emergency, I must act quickly to keep your wife and babies safe."*

A pause. Then, his shoulders relaxed. *"I understand,"* he finally said. And then, the joy returned. He turned to his wife, the three babies nestled around her, and his expression softened into pure elation.

A Hard Conversation

Having passed the critical 34-week mark, the babies were stable enough to avoid the NICU. The pediatric team offered standard newborn care: hepatitis B vaccines, vitamin K, and formula supplementation. Jared and his wife declined everything, determined to keep things as natural as possible.

The next day, I returned to check on them. I was still riding the high of the previous night's success—triplets delivered vaginally, a first for our hospital. It felt like a victory for this familys autonomy and natural birth.

But as I sat down to chart, several urgent notices flashed across my screen. Two nurses approached me, their faces drawn with worry.

"Something's wrong," one of them said. *"You need to see this."*

I read the notes. My eyes widened. My jaw hit the keyboard.

I turned to the nurses. *"Did I just read what I think I read?"*

The senior nurse nodded gravely. *"Yes."*

Jared's wife, still struggling with narcolepsy, had fallen asleep while holding Baby A and dropped the newborn onto the hospital floor.

Jared had rushed to scoop up the baby, hitting the call button in a panic. The pediatric team arrived, assessed the baby, and—again—offered vitamin K.

Again, they refused.

The nurses were beside themselves. *"Doctor,"* one said, *"These babies had a tough delivery. Baby B was breech, a higher risk for hemorrhage. Baby C needed vacuum extraction—potential bruising and internal bleeding. And now this fall..."*

I exhaled sharply. They were right. All three babies had an increased risk of internal bleeding, and without vitamin K, they were vulnerable.

I made my way to their room for one final conversation. Would they listen? Could I convince them before it was too late?

Baby in the Pants—A Story of Autonomy

Cherise was a highly educated professor, married to another professor at a distinguished university in Arizona. When she first came to me, she was in search of co-care for her pregnancy, though it was clear she was only there because her Midwife insisted.

From the moment she walked in, she made her stance clear.

"My Midwife wants me to have co-care with you, Dr. Hervey, but I do not want to see you."

I smiled, unfazed. I'd heard variations of this before.

"I'm not here to tell you what to do," I reassured her. *"I'm here to provide you with options so you can decide what's best for your body, your baby, and your family. My job is never to force or coerce you. That would be assault. My job is to educate."*

I reminded her that she was an educated woman, highly educated. And educated people make informed decisions.

The introduction ended on a civil note, and we proceeded with the routine evaluations. At that stage, early in the first trimester, she was low-risk—early 30s, low BMI, healthy, and highly motivated. We agreed to see each other once a month throughout her pregnancy unless concerns arose.

Month after month, everything remained stable. Then, somewhere along the way, she stopped coming. Perhaps she no longer saw the need, and instead relied solely on her midwife.

Then, at 36 weeks, she was back on my schedule.

She sat before me, her frustration palpable.

"I don't want to be here," she stated, glaring. "*I want to have my home birth."*

I glanced at her chart. Blood pressure:140s–150s over 90s.

Her Midwife had noted elevated readings and had strongly advised her to return under my care. I laid out the facts and offered a full preeclampsia workup. Reluctantly, she agreed to the labs, but refused any hypertensive medication.

"I'll manage it myself," she insisted. *"Lower stress, better diet, lifestyle changes."*

I provided a blood pressure log and a cuff so she could track her readings at home. I gave her clear guidelines: If your blood pressure reaches 160/110, you must go directly to the hospital.

A week later, she returned. Blood pressure: 150/100.

I urged her to start a low-dose beta-blocker to help her maintain a stable pregnancy and avoid induction. She refused induction outright but begrudgingly agreed to the medication. At this point, she could no longer be considered a candidate for home birth.

She wasn't happy about it, but she understood.

Then, she vanished again.

She missed her next appointment. My nurse called to check in.

Her response was simple:

"Every time I come in, there's bad news. So, I decided I wasn't coming in anymore."

Dangerous logic.

I called her myself. I reiterated everything we had already discussed.

"The Greek definition of Preeclampsia is lightning; it happens quickly and with fury". "Preeclampsia is like storm clouds on the side of the highway," I explained. *"It is dark, angry clouds on the*

horizon. You see them, but there's no rain yet. You know the storm is coming, but you think: Can I make it home before it hits?" "Then lightning strikes, seizures or a stroke".

Doctors, like experienced travelers, see the storm for what it is. We don't wait for the downpour. We take shelter—medications, monitoring, interventions—before the storm strikes.

She apologized for missing the appointment. Promised to come to the next one. But she still wasn't ready for induction.

Her at-home readings? 140s, sometimes 150s. Stuck in the 90s.

Then, at 38 weeks and five days, she showed up at the hospital.

Her water had broken. She claimed to be in labor. She wasn't.

Blood pressure: 160s–170s, occasionally 180s.

Still, no symptoms—no headaches, no vision changes. The baby looked good on the monitor. But she was adamant about natural labor. She refused Pitocin. Refused magnesium sulfate to prevent seizures and strokes.

Her husband, an intellectual himself, was torn between frustration and support. He understood the risks—and so did she. But she remained resolute.

I kept offering magnesium. She kept declining.

Two days passed. She was still not in labor.

She accepted nifedipine to control her blood pressure but continued to refuse any interventions that would induce labor. I called Maternal-Fetal Medicine and other OB colleagues, hoping they could convince her.

Nothing changed.

Day three and a half.

Exhausted and frustrated, her husband left the hospital to feed the dogs.

"She hasn't had a seizure," he told me before he left. *"She hasn't had a stroke. The baby looks fine."*

He was rationalizing. It hadn't happened yet, so maybe it wouldn't.

Inside, Cherise was trying every natural method to induce labor—breast pumps, movement, and position changes. Nothing worked.

She refused exams, so we still didn't know how dilated she was.

She wore her street clothes the entire time.

Finally, after over three days, she relented.

"Fine."

Two units of Pitocin. Just for 30 minutes.

Her contractions kicked in. We turned the Pitocin off.

And then—we waited.

Four hours later, I was called to her room.

She was writhing, rolling, and moaning.

She was still wearing her pants.

"I need to push!" She screamed.

She never took off her pants. The baby was born into her pants.

Her husband returned to find her with their newborn on her chest—relieved, triumphant.

I offered magnesium again, standard care to prevent seizures and strokes.

She declined.

Both she and the baby were stable. She agreed to stay one extra day for postpartum observation due to her severe blood pressure readings.

In the end, she got the birth she wanted. And I got the ending I feared, but was grateful it didn't happen. A win for autonomy, a gamble against preeclampsia, and a baby in the pants.

These stories—*Birth on the Brink*, *Baby in the Pants*, and *Birth Against the Odds*—each present complex moral dilemmas that Obstetrical providers frequently face when working with non-traditional families or patients who challenge standard medical recommendations. The themes that emerge from these narratives offer valuable insights into autonomy, provider-patient trust, and the ethics of balancing medical responsibility with patient choice.

Moral Dilemmas in Obstetric Care: Navigating the Edge of Autonomy and Advocacy

Obstetric care exists at the crossroads of medical science, human emotion, and moral complexity. It is one of the few clinical arenas where the stakes are high for two lives, and yet the locus of control remains deeply personal. In this space, we confront moral dilemmas not as rare exceptions, but as the daily rhythm of practice.

1. Autonomy vs. Medical Responsibility

Each difficult case brings us face-to-face with the tension between a patients right to autonomy and our professional obligation to protect life and prevent harm. What happens when a patient refuses an intervention that could prevent seizure, stroke, or death? What is our role when we foresee a catastrophe, but they choose otherwise?

- Where is the ethical line between honoring autonomy and abandoning responsibility?

- At what point does autonomy veer into negligence, and who has the right to draw that line?

Take *Cherise*—the unforgettable case of *Baby in the Pants*. She had the intellectual capacity to comprehend the escalating risks of preeclampsia. She was fully informed. Yet, as her blood pressure crept higher and her risk of seizure increased, she consistently declined interventions. From a legal standpoint, her choices were protected. From a medical perspective, they were perilously irrational.

Our ethical grounding must be strongest in this tension between medical foresight and patient rights. The team's coordinated response—carefully documenting discussions, persistently offering support, and aligning staff on tone and messaging—was essential. We did not coerce. We communicated clearly, compassionately, and consistently. And though her labor path was harrowing, it ended in safety, not because we controlled it, but because we stayed present within the chaos.

2. Risk Perception vs. Risk Reality

Some patients believe that understanding risk is the same as neutralizing it. In our data-driven age, education can give patients a false sense of security, as if naming a condition somehow immunizes them against it.

In *Birth Against the Odds*, the family's conviction in natural birth overrode even the most glaring warning signs. In *Baby in the Pants*, Cherise behaved as if simply knowing about preeclampsia would render it powerless.

But knowledge does not override physiology.

As providers, one of our core tasks is bridging the gap between what patients *know* and what they *feel*. I often use storytelling here, not as manipulation, but as a deeply human form of education. When a patient minimizes a serious condition, I recall the case of a 28-week mom who had no elevated pressures during her pregnancy. She went to the mall one afternoon, shopping with her sisters, and collapsed in a seizure. Her stroke came like lightning—sudden, violent, and without warning.

I describe preeclampsia to patients as a gathering storm. The skies may look clear, but the wind is changing. The pressure is dropping. You may not see it, but those of us trained to read the horizon know it's coming. And when it hits, it doesn't negotiate.

Stories and analogies convert abstract data into living truths. They help patients recognize that risk isn't just a number—it's a presence, and sometimes, a predator.

3. When Beliefs and Culture Challenge Medical Norms

Many families enter childbirth with deep cultural values or long-standing skepticism toward the medical system. They may prioritize home birth, reject pharmaceuticals, or cling to spiritual or holistic beliefs that sit at odds with hospital protocol.

Our role is not to "correct" these views but to navigate them with empathy and intellectual humility.

A Medical ICU nurse and Advanced Nurse Practitioner student recently asked for a lotus birth during a scheduled cesarean. Her baby was breech at 41 weeks, with no labor signs and a foot presenting. She and her home birth Midwife had attempted four versions of external cephalic rotation. None succeeded. The baby was macrocosmic, and vaginal birth was no longer safe. She was devastated—but determined to preserve the sanctity of her birth vision.

We met her where she was. In compromise, we performed a lotus birth by cesarean. She held onto her placenta long after delivery, asking repeatedly if it had turned white, a sign she believed indicated separation readiness. Despite her clinical training, it was clear her understanding was filtered more through ideology than biology.

This case taught me something: beliefs often endure even when evidence is available. Our job is to find the human within the belief—to build trust, not confront it head-on with condescension. Even in disagreement, we must leave room for dignity.

4. The Role of the Provider: Educator, Guardian, or Enforcer?

Obstetric providers must constantly shift roles in response to dynamic patient needs and crises:

- The educator shares knowledge and trusts patients to make decisions—even when they choose the riskier path.
- The Guardian advocates strongly while still respecting autonomy.
- The Enforcer invokes legal tools or institutional authority when life is imminently at risk and consent is withheld.

Most of us aspire to be Educators. It's the most collaborative, the most humane. But when seconds count, and a uterus is rupturing or an eclamptic seizure is beginning, the Guardian can quickly transform into the Enforcer.

It is a moral calculus that offers no easy answers. Each case demands a reckoning with one's own boundaries. As clinicians, we must ask: *When does my moral obligation override patient preference? And am I willing to live with that choice?*

Practical Wisdom: Working with Challenging or Non-Traditional Families

1. Lead with Curiosity, Not Judgment

When a patient resists, it's tempting to become defensive or dismissive. Instead, lean in with curiosity.

- *What are they afraid of?*
- *Where does their belief come from?*
- *Is it mistrust, trauma, cultural identity, or misinformed confidence?*

With *Habid and Sophia*, understanding their cultural context helped resolve a communication impasse that no number of statistics could touch. Listening is a diagnostic skill—use it often.

2. Make Risk Feel Real, Not Just Logical

People don't change their behavior because of numbers. They change when risk becomes emotionally visible.

- Use analogies, not just algorithms.
- Make the invisible threat feel tangible—something they can see and grasp.

- Remind them that *being the exception* is a seductive myth. Everyone believes theyre the one who 'll be fine—until they're not.

3. Negotiate, Don't Dictate

Top-down commands rarely work in Obstetrics. Negotiation does.

- Offer flexible options within safe limits.
- Use language that empowers: "I want to work with you," not "You have to."
- Respect bodily autonomy always: "No one should do anything to you without your consent. Ever."

In *Baby in the Pants*, Cherise rejected almost every intervention. But through mutual respect and clear boundaries, we reached an agreement on low-dose Pitocin—enough to progress her labor without betraying her wishes.

4. Expect—and Embrace—the Unconventional

Birth is wild, creative, and untamed. So are patients.

You might see a baby delivered while the mother stands upright, pants still on. You might meet a family who declines every postpartum medication—and still walks out with a healthy child.

Success in Obstetrics isn't defined by strict adherence to a plan. It's defined by whether we offered safety, dignity, and compassion—even when the birth was nothing like we imagined.

That's what saved Lisa's and Johanna's babies.

Medicine as a Partnership, Not a Dictatorship

Obstetrics is not a field of control. It's a discipline of stewardship. Of partnership. Of reading the wind and knowing when to steer and when to surrender.

Some patients will fight the storm. Some will misjudge its danger. Some will test our ethics, stretch our empathy, and defy our protocols. And sometimes, yes, a baby will be born into their mother's pants.

This is not failure. It is the raw, unpredictable, deeply human work we chose.

And if we do it right—with presence, patience, and principle-we, we dont just deliver babies. We deliver dignity, even in dissent. We become not only providers of care, but practitioners of wisdom.

Jade's Story

Jade arrived at our clinic at 28 weeks pregnant. She had been planning a home birth with a well-respected Midwife in the community. At just 24 years old, newly married, and expecting her first child, she was filled with joy and excitement about the life growing inside her. But when she stepped into our clinic, she was in tears. Her world had just shattered. She had been diagnosed with stage four inflammatory breast cancer. They were lost, unsure of what to do, desperately seeking medical advice at the highest level.

Jade had envisioned a long life with her husband and their newborn baby. Now, that dream was rocked by the fear of an incurable disease. She struggled with the idea of introducing powerful chemotherapy drugs into her body—medications that could affect her baby's health, not just now but in the future.

This is where I met Jade.

She had initially been ecstatic about her pregnancy, having met with her home birth Midwife early on, eager for the journey ahead. At one of her routine visits, she had casually mentioned a lump in her breast. The Midwife examined it and reassured her, *"It's probably nothing. Let's keep an eye on it, and if it changes, we can look into it further after you have your baby. Just focus on the pregnancy."*

Jade, young and naive to the dangers, trusted this guidance. She continued her pregnancy without much concern, even as the lump persisted. Over time, she noticed slight changes—twinges of pain, discomfort when wearing a bra, and a growing sensitivity during intimacy. She brought it up again at another visit, and this time, the Midwife ordered imaging. A mammogram led to an ultrasound the same day, followed by an immediate consultation with a radiologist who urgently requested a biopsy. The results were devastating—stage four inflammatory breast cancer, already spreading to her lymph nodes.

The Midwife, in a panic, reached out to me. She reviewed the diagnostic reports with me and asked if I would assume Jade's care. That's how I found myself sitting in front of Jade and her husband, trying to help them navigate an impossible decision. I had so many questions, empathetically, curious —if this mass had been evaluated when she first mentioned it, would we have caught it earlier? Would she have had better options? Had it been diagnosed in the first trimester, perhaps she and her husband would have chosen to focus on her treatment. But now, in the third trimester, there was no choice. It was no longer about choosing between mother and baby. We had to fight for both. My mind raced as far as to ask, have I ever missed the opportunity to diagnose a devastating diagnosis? This could have been any one of my many patients; any one of us.

The oncologists were ready to begin chemotherapy immediately. But Jade, so devoted to her baby, was hesitant. She was willing to endure anything if it meant protecting her child. I contacted a close friend, the CEO of a major cancer center, to ensure she received the best possible care. She underwent the highest level of evaluation and consultation. But her cancer was aggressive.

She started feeling unwell and was admitted to the hospital for severe anemia and fatigue. After three days, she was discharged, but she was a shadow of the woman I had first met. A week or two later, she was hospitalized again—this time, gravely ill. At 35–36 weeks pregnant, Maternal-Fetal Medicine stepped in. The recommendation was clear: deliver the baby so that Jade could begin aggressive treatment immediately.

She had a beautiful, unmedicated labor, induced with the help of my favorite Midwife- my wife. She and her baby went home together, cherishing their little time as a family.

Jade received her first round of chemotherapy. It ravaged her body. She was hospitalized again and never left. She passed away about ten weeks after giving birth.

Jade's Autonomous Dilemma

Jade's story is one of profound courage and heartbreaking complexity. Her late-stage cancer diagnosis came after weeks of reassuring assessments, during which she placed her trust in the care she was receiving. By the time she was referred for specialized evaluation, her options had narrowed.

When the recommendation came to begin chemotherapy during pregnancy, Jade was faced with an impossible choice: prioritize her own aggressive treatment or protect the life growing inside her. She chose, as many mothers might, to focus on her baby's well-being, hoping to buy time, to preserve possibility.

Her medical team shared their concerns openly and compassionately. Yet Jade's values—her identity as a mother, her hopes for her child—guided her decisions. She held tightly to her autonomy, even as the risks mounted.

Jade passed shortly after childbirth. Her story is not one of fault, but of the heartbreaking tension between two sacred lives. It reminds us that autonomy does not exist in a vacuum; it is shaped by the information available, the timing of diagnoses, and the emotional weight of decisions no one should ever have to make.

In honoring her journey, we're reminded of the delicate balance we walk as providers—to inform without overwhelming, support without steering, and hold space for life and loss with equal reverence.

Tonya's Story

Tonya walked into my office at 12 weeks pregnant, accompanied by her fiancé, mother, and sister. The small exam room was packed. Her fiancé was a noticeable presence, towering at six feet two with broad shoulders and long dreadlocks. Tonya, though not small herself, looked tiny beside him.

They were excited to meet me, having heard great things about my care philosophy. But there was also an unspoken heaviness in the air. When an entire family shows up for an early prenatal visit, there's usually more beneath the surface—a complex situation, a challenge that needs to be navigated.

For Tonya, that challenge was breast cancer.

Diagnosed nearly simultaneously with her pregnancy, she had a small, isolated lump in her right breast. Her original OB immediately recommended termination, followed by surgical and chemotherapy treatment. Maternal-Fetal Medicine echoed the same advice. Every OB she saw gave her the same recommendation: abort the pregnancy, undergo treatment, and preserve her chances of having children in the future.

Medically, it was sound advice. The cancer was small but aggressive. With treatment, her prognosis was strong. But to Tonya and her devout Christian family, abortion was never an option.

Her faith was unwavering. She believed she would be healed through prayer, dietary changes, and holistic remedies. She wore crosses on her jewelry, tattoos, and clothing—reminders of the hope she refused to relinquish.

I approached our conversation as I did with all my patients and promised to continue reminding her of the medical standards, not to pressure her, but to ensure she made an informed choice. She agreed. Her family agreed.

We monitored her closely, ensuring both she and the baby remained stable. At 28 weeks, we conducted a routine glucose test. And then—she disappeared.

For nearly two months, I heard nothing. No calls, no visits. At 36 weeks, we had no idea where she was. Had she switched providers? Had her condition worsened? My medical assistant called her, urging her to come in.

When she finally arrived, she looked well. She is still adorned with her faith-based attire, hopeful and trusting in her path. But she was exhausted, emotionally drained from constantly hearing about risk and mortality. *"I'm tired of the same conversation,"* she admitted. *"I feel good. My baby is doing great. My faith is strong. I just want to enjoy this pregnancy."*

I pleaded with her to see Maternal-Fetal Medicine for a final evaluation and to consult with oncology. She agreed. But when she returned, her reality had shifted. The cancer had grown. It had spread. It was worse.

At 37 weeks, her family begged me to help her deliver. *"Doctor, can we have our baby?"*

She went into labor naturally. A smooth, uncomplicated vaginal birth- VBAC.

She was discharged within 24 hours.

Six weeks later, she returned for her postpartum visit. She looked different—thin and pale, with a baseball cap covering her bald head. But she was alive. She had undergone surgery, started chemotherapy, and was preparing for radiation.

A year later, I received an invitation—a wedding invitation.

Tonya was marrying her fiancé. And inside was a picture of their baby boy.

Both Jade and Tonya faced profound dilemmas centered on autonomy in healthcare, particularly in the context of pregnancy and life-threatening illness. Their situations highlight the tension between medical recommendations, personal values, and the right to make informed decisions about one's own body.

Tonya's Autonomous Dilemma

Tonya's dilemma was different but equally complex. Diagnosed early in pregnancy, she was given a clear medical recommendation: terminate the pregnancy to pursue aggressive cancer treatment. However, her deeply held religious beliefs made abortion non-negotiable. Unlike Jade, Tonya had the opportunity to exercise autonomy from the outset, fully aware of her diagnosis and the risks involved. She chose faith-based healing over immediate medical intervention despite continued medical warnings. Her autonomy was also challenged when she disengaged from care, seeking relief from the constant pressure of medical advice. In the end, she survived, but her journey was defined by her assertion of control over her body, even when it defied medical recommendations.

Their stories illustrate how autonomy in healthcare is not absolute but is influenced by timing, access to information, values, and systemic pressures.

Amy's Story

Amy was an intriguing patient, petite, of Caribbean descent, with deep roots in African heritage. Her partner, tall and lanky, was African American. They eagerly expected their first child and envisioned a natural birth. They had chosen Midwifery care from the beginning, embracing a medication-free, intervention-free experience. They even planned a lotus birth, where the placenta remains attached to the baby until it naturally separates.

At around 38 weeks, Amy was sent to the hospital to meet me. A newly developed arrhythmia had been detected at a routine clinic appointment two weeks prior. She had already seen a specialist, who strongly recommended immediate delivery due to the atypical nature of the arrhythmia. The irregular heartbeat was initially suspected to be caused by fetal heart cells firing inconsistently. But after prolonged monitoring, a different pattern emerged—one that was alarming. The baby's heart rate would slow to match the mother's, dropping into the 70s and 80s, before climbing back to a baseline of 120–130 bpm, repeating in cycles.

Despite a reassuring biophysical profile, something didn't sit right. Over the following weeks, the condition became more persistent. The Midwife, growing increasingly concerned, performed Doppler assessments and worried the baby could be experiencing distress. She strongly urged Amy to go to the hospital for delivery.

As soon as Amy arrived on the labor floor, alarms went off. The moment we placed her on the monitor, we saw repetitive drops in the baby's heart rate, dipping low and then recovering. This happened three times an hour, sometimes stabilizing for long stretches before occurring again. The fetal echocardiogram appeared normal aside from the erratic heart rate, but Maternal-Fetal Medicine was concerned. They recommended delivery, and not just any delivery, but a C-section. The unpredictable heart rate patterns made continuous monitoring unreliable, and the inability to differentiate between benign arrhythmias and dangerous decelerations posed a serious risk.

But Amy was resolute. *"I do not want a C-section,"* she said. *"I want a natural birth. I want a lotus birth. No medications, no interventions."*

Everything she had planned was unraveling, and she was unwilling to compromise. Her family gathered at her bedside. The Midwife and doula sat with us. I spoke to her as I always do, with transparency and respect. "You are the boss, and I am here to provide options. You decide." I outlined the dangers. If the baby's heart rate dropped and we couldn't tell whether it was a harmless arrhythmia or a true emergency, we might rush into a C-section unnecessarily. Worse, the outcome could be devastating if we misjudged the situation and failed to act when needed.

For five days, we talked, educated, and consulted. We brought in family, specialists, and ethics committees. But Amy did not waver. *"I understand the risks,"* she said. *"I still choose natural birth."*

Every day, we monitored the baby's biophysical profile. Every day, the same thing happened concerning heart rate dips. But the baby held steady. And so we waited.

On the eighth day, Amy went into spontaneous labor. She was 3cm dilated and contracting regularly. It was time.

We had to navigate her labor carefully. She agreed to spot monitoring but refused continuous tracing. We all breathed, praying the baby's heart would hold firm.

Four hours in, her water broke. An hour later, she began to push.

With no interventions, no pain medication, and against all odds, Amy delivered a healthy baby.

She had fought for the birth she wanted. And she had won.

The Autonomy Dilemma in Amy's Story

Amy's case presented one of the most challenging dilemmas I have faced as a provider—the conflict between respecting a patient's autonomy and ensuring the best possible outcome for her baby.

She was competent, well-informed, and unwavering in her decision. Despite clear medical concerns, including an unpredictable fetal arrhythmia that made it nearly impossible to differentiate normal fluctuations from life-threatening decelerations, she refused a C-section. She had a vision for her birth, and no amount of medical reasoning, consultations, or risk assessments would change her mind.

I found myself caught between two ethical obligations: honoring her right to make decisions about her body and ensuring the safety of her unborn child. My medical training and instincts urged me to act and intervene before the situation became critical. However, Amy understood the risks, verbalized them clearly, and was determined to proceed on her terms.

This left me and the entire medical team with limited options. We could not override her autonomy without legal or ethical justification, neither of which was present. Instead, we had to find a way to navigate this rigid refusal while minimizing risk.

Navigating a Rigid Patient Refusing Recommended Care

When a patient refuses care that a provider deems medically necessary, several steps can be taken to navigate the situation effectively:

1. Thorough Education and Informed Consent

- I ensured Amy understood the medical risks in detail, using clear explanations and repeated discussions over several days.
- I provided real-world examples and case studies to illustrate possible outcomes.
- I emphasized that our goal was not to pressure her but to ensure she had all the facts before deciding.

2. Multidisciplinary Consultation

- Specialists, including Maternal-Fetal Medicine, cardiology, and neonatology, were brought in to assess the situation and provide their recommendations.

- Hospital ethics and legal teams were consulted to ensure we acted within the boundaries of medical ethics and the law.

3. Engaging Family and Support Systems

- I encouraged discussions with her partner, family members, and her doula.
- Sometimes, hearing the same information from a trusted loved one can help a patient reconsider their stance.

4. Compromise and Shared Decision-Making

- Rather than an all-or-nothing approach, I worked with Amy to find a middle ground.
- She agreed to spot monitoring instead of continuous monitoring, which allowed us to keep some level of fetal assessment without violating her birth plan entirely.
- We established a clear emergency protocol in case immediate intervention became necessary.

5. Careful Documentation

- Every discussion, every risk explained, and every decision made by Amy was meticulously documented.

- This was crucial not only for legal protection but also to ensure transparency in the shared decision-making process.

6. Respecting Autonomy While Remaining Prepared

- Though I firmly believed a C-section was the safest option, I had to respect Amy's decision.

- My focus shifted to monitoring, adjusting care within her boundaries, and being prepared to act immediately in an emergency.

Ultimately, Amy gave birth exactly as she had envisioned—without interventions, without pain medication, and on her terms. It was a rare resolution where autonomy and medical safety coexisted, but it required patience, communication, and a willingness to navigate the complexities of shared decision-making.

In the end, Amy's case reinforced a fundamental truth in medicine: our role is not to dictate care but to guide, support, and, when necessary, stand by a patient's choices—even when they go against everything we have been trained to do.

Autonomy in patient care does not mean agreement. It does not mean the provider endorses the patient's choices, hopes, or wishes. Instead, autonomy is the provider's willingness to step back and let the patient take the lead, while still guiding them, offering knowledge, and standing ready to intervene if necessary.

Caring for a patient is like teaching a child to ride a bike. Throughout pregnancy, we ensure the training wheels are secure at every visit, running alongside them and sharing what is standard, safe, and best practice. The patient pedals freely, gaining confidence with each decision. Occasionally, we reach out, steadying the handlebars to keep them upright.

Then comes labor—the day those training wheels come off. The provider stands beside them, launching them forward and running alongside them as they wobble. The more they trust us, the more they trust themselves. The distance between us widens. Most of the time, they ride independently and confidently. But sometimes, they fall. And when they do, we are there to pick them up, to dust them off, and to help them decide: Do we put the training wheels back on, or do we allow them to learn from the fall and try again?

Margaret's Story

Margaret was like many of my patients—advanced maternal age, conceived through IVF, but deeply committed to a natural birth experience. She sought care from a doula and a home-birth Midwife, stepping away from hospital-based medicine entirely. At 45, she was remarkably healthy, thin, with a low BMI, no diabetes, and no hypertension. But hospitals made her feel vulnerable. She didn't trust them. She didn't feel safe. And so, she left my care.

Then, at 41 weeks and six days, Margaret arrived at the hospital. She was in latent labor; her water had broken. In the triage room, she stood rocking back and forth, refusing monitoring, refusing an exam. Yet, the report from her Midwife was deeply concerning—there had been prolonged, deep decelerations in the baby's heart rate, a sign of fetal distress.

The resident, Ben, approached her first. He was kind, patient, and skilled. He offered an exam, a moment to listen to the baby, anything that would give us a clue as to how her baby was tolerating labor. But Margaret had one request: she wanted to be transferred to a labor room, to get in the tub, and then—perhaps—she would allow monitoring and an exam.

I stepped in and told her the risks and what was at stake.

I looked at her, this strong, determined woman who had fought so hard to have this baby, who had carefully built a plan to bring them into the world on her terms. I knew what this birth meant to her. But I also knew what the data was telling us.

"Margaret," I said gently. *"We are concerned about you. We are concerned about your baby."*

I explained what we knew—that meconium in the amniotic fluid could indicate distress, that it was rare for a 45-year-old patient to maintain pregnancy until 41 weeks, that standard guidelines for advanced maternal age recommended delivery at 39 weeks, and that for IVF pregnancies, 40 weeks was the safest cutoff. I reminded her that she had worked so hard to conceive this child, to have a healthy baby, to have a safe delivery. And we wanted to help her achieve those things.

After some time, she agreed to an exam.

Her cervix was high, thick, and only 2cm dilated—she was nowhere near delivery. And then, when she lay down, and we placed the monitors, we saw it:

Every contraction, every four minutes, the baby's heart rate dropped into the 60s.

We had no way of knowing how long this had been happening. But we knew what it meant. This was ominous.

I took a deep breath and said, *"Margaret, your baby is unhappy. Your baby is losing oxygen. Your baby is in distress."*

I tried to frame it in a way she could accept. I used my airplane analogy to help. *"We are on a flight, and on this flight, we have hit turbulence. Like most flight turbulence occurs at two times, taking off and landing. Landing, we often can push through and land at our desired destination. Taking off is more challenging because we don't know how long our flight will ultimately be. Flying from Phoenix to San Francisco is a very short 45-minute flight; I would support you continuing on the same path, and we will land at our destination and how we desire. But if we're flying to Japan, and the turbulence is severe, we might have to change course to land somewhere else, somewhere safe."*

I looked at her. *"We have a long way to go for a vaginal birth. But your baby is telling us they can't take this journey."*

Still, she resisted. For over an hour, we went back and forth—her desire for a natural birth warring against the stark reality of what was unfolding. Repeat cervical check showed no change.

Finally, she agreed. We rushed her to the OR for an emergency C-section.

The outcome? A live baby, but profoundly compromised. They spent over 30 days in the NICU.

Margaret had fought for her autonomy and won, until biology, nature, and the undeniable truth of labor took over. Ultimately, the right decision was made, but at a cost.

This is the delicate, fragile dance of autonomy in patient care. It is the balance between respect and responsibility, between choice and consequence. It is knowing when to let the patient pedal freely, and when to reach out and grab the handlebars before they fall.

Margaret's story presents a classic autonomy dilemma, where her desire for independence clashes with the responsibilities and consequences of her choices. As she strives to assert control over her life, she faces difficult decisions that impact her and those around her. Her pursuit of autonomy may lead to unintended consequences, such as strained relationships, personal sacrifice, or even regret if her choices do not align with her long-term well-being. At the same time, surrendering her independence to external influences—whether societal expectations, family pressure, or financial constraints—could result in a loss of self-identity and personal fulfillment. Ultimately, Margaret's journey highlights the complex balance between self-determination and the inevitable repercussions of the paths we choose to take.

Respecting a woman's autonomy in decision-making while ensuring she is fully informed about the risks and benefits of each option is essential. The healthcare provider's role is not to dictate decisions but to educate and offer options, while also knowing when intervention is necessary to protect the well-being of both mother and baby and the delicate balance of providing support while acknowledging the challenges that can arise during pregnancy and birth, highlighting both the complexities of medical decisions and the importance of a compassionate approach to patient care.

Conclusion

The take-home message of *"Her Body, Her Baby"* is the power and complexity of patient autonomy in medical care, especially in Obstetrics, where two lives are at stake. It highlights how informed decision-making, mutual respect, and shared responsibility between provider and patient create the foundation for ethical, compassionate, and safe medical practice.

Through real-world examples like April's, the text underscores that autonomy does not mean patients reject medical expertise, nor should doctors relinquish their duty to provide guidance. Instead, it is about bridging the gap, ensuring patients understand risks and options while allowing them to maintain control over their bodies and births.

We as providers exist to be that soft landing—a place where patient autonomy is honored, guided by educated support. We provide more than just medical care. We offer a sense of humanism, recognizing the whole person, the whole patient, and the complex, layered experiences each individual brings to their birth journey.

One of my favorite examples of this was with Rochelle.

Rochelle had previously had four home births and only came to our practice because her baby had been diagnosed with a cardiac defect that would require surgery immediately after birth. She was clear from the beginning: she wanted an experience as close as possible to what she had in her home births. Because of that, it was natural to connect her with one of the Midwives in our practice.

When Rochelle came to the hospital in labor, we ensured all the necessary medical preparations were made. The children's hospital was notified, the NICU team was on standby, and the cardiac surgeon was alerted. Although Rochelles delivery itself was expected to be uncomplicated, I was present as surgical backup—an example of true collaborative care.

Then came a twist. The NICU team requested that Rochelle deliver in the operating room because all their high-risk tools and materials were located there. Rochelle was in active labor, 9.5 cm dilated, starting to feel the urge to push. She didn't want to be wheeled on a stretcher—she wanted to walk. So she walked herself from the labor unit to the OR.

Once in the OR, the staff had set up the standard operating table with stirrups, expecting her to lie down and push. Rochelle took one look at it and said, crystal clear, *"I'm not getting on that. I don't need that."*

The Midwife looked at her and agreed. Then they both looked at me, the most senior person in the room. I said, *"I agree. There's nothing wrong with this mother."*

I turned to Rochelle and asked, *"What would you like?"* Without hesitation, she answered, *"I'd like to stand up and push my baby out. That's what I've done in the past."*

So we adapted. The OR table was pushed aside, a stack of warm blankets was placed on the floor under the radiant warmer, and Rochelle stood, leaning over the OR table. The Midwife knelt, ready to receive the baby. Rochelle bore down—and it was a beautiful, uneventful delivery.

After about a minute and a half of delayed cord clamping, the cord was cut, and the baby was passed to the NICU team for evaluation. Rochelle then used the OR table only so we could assist in delivering the placenta. That was it.

What Rochelle needed wasn't complicated. She needed safety. She needed control. She needed to feel heard.

And one of the simplest, most common things patients ask—often just as Rochelle did—is: *"Do I have to push on my back?"*

It seems so basic, but in the world of modern Obstetrics—where protocols often override preferences—that question can be a quiet act of resistance. Too many providers insist, demand, or lack flexibility on how a woman gives birth.

Rochelle's story is a testament to what happens when we listen. She had a safe birth in a hospital, on her terms, with the team ready for any emergency. That's what she needed—a soft landing.

Since then, countless friends of Rochelle from college and beyond have come to us when they needed support. Rochelle herself returned to deliver her next baby in the hospital—not because she had to, but because she knew she would be supported. She trusted us because we saw her.

For providers, the message is clear: We are not the decision-makers; we are the facilitators of informed choices. The best care is not about enforcing protocols but fostering trust and partnership, even when a patient's decision challenges conventional medical recommendations.

For patients, autonomy affirms their right to be heard and respected in their healthcare decisions, proving that a well-informed and unwavering voice can shape outcomes that honor medical knowledge and personal values.

Ultimately, *"Her Body, Her Baby"* is a testament to the delicate balance between medical ethics, autonomy, and providers profound responsibility to ensure safety and respect in the birth process. This is a movement for change!

EXAMPLE COMMUNICATIONS:

Glossary

Acceleration: A temporary increase in fetal heart rate, generally considered a sign of fetal well-being.

AGA (Appropriate for Gestational Age): Describes a fetus or newborn whose size is within the normal range for their gestational age, typically between the 10th and 90th percentiles.

AMA (Advanced Maternal Age): Refers to pregnant individuals who are 35 years or older at the expected delivery time.

AMA (Against Medical Advice): When a patient chooses to leave or discontinue medical care despite their healthcare providers recommendations.

AROM (Artificial Rupture of Membranes): A medical procedure where the amniotic sac is deliberately ruptured to induce or accelerate labor.

BMI (Body Mass Index): A measure of body fat based on an individuals weight relative to their height, used to categorize underweight, normal weight, overweight, and obesity.

Breech: A fetal position where the baby is positioned to deliver buttocks or feet first instead of the head.

Category 1 Fetal Heart Tracing: A classification indicating standard fetal heart rate patterns, suggesting the fetus is well-oxygenated.

Category 2 Fetal Heart Tracing: A classification indicating indeterminate fetal heart rate patterns that do not predict abnormal fetal acid-base status.

Category 3 Fetal Heart Tracing: A classification indicating abnormal fetal heart rate patterns, suggesting the fetus may be in distress and may require immediate intervention.

Cephalic: A fetal position where the babys head is positioned downward in the uterus, typically considered the optimal position for vaginal delivery.

Deceleration: A temporary decrease in fetal heart rate, which can be benign or indicate potential fetal distress, depending on the pattern and timing.

Di-Di Twins (Dichorionic-Diamniotic Twins): Twins with separate chorions and amniotic sacs can occur in identical and fraternal twins.

FGR (Fetal Growth Restriction): A condition where a fetus is unable to achieve its genetically determined potential size, often defined as an estimated fetal weight below the 10th percentile for gestational age.

First Trimester: The initial stage of pregnancy, spanning from conception to 12 weeks of gestation.

Forceps: A surgical instrument resembling a pair of tongs used to assist in delivering a baby by grasping the babys head.

Gravida: The number of times a person has been pregnant, regardless of the outcome.

IUGR (Intrauterine Growth Restriction): Another term for fetal growth restriction, indicating poor growth of a fetus while in the mothers womb during pregnancy.

IVF (In Vitro Fertilization): An assisted reproductive technology where an egg is fertilized by sperm outside the body, and the resulting embryo is implanted into the uterus.

Macrosomia: A condition where a fetus has an estimated weight of more than 4,000 grams (8 pounds, 13 ounces), regardless of gestational age.

Maternal Mortality: The death of a woman during pregnancy, childbirth, or within 42 days of delivery, irrespective of the duration and site of the pregnancy, from any cause related to or aggravated by the pregnancy or its management.

Mono-Di Twins (Monochorionic-Diamniotic Twins): Identical twins that share the same chorion (outer membrane) but have separate amniotic sacs.

Pelvic Floor Dysfunction is when the muscles and tissues supporting the pelvic organs weaken or are injured, leading to issues like incontinence or prolapse.

Placenta Abruption: A condition where the placenta detaches from the uterine wall before delivery, which can deprive the fetus of oxygen and nutrients.

Placenta Previa: A condition where the placenta partially or wholly covers the cervix, potentially causing severe bleeding during pregnancy and delivery.

Post-Operatively: Refers to the period after a surgical operation.

Pre-Eclampsia: A pregnancy complication characterized by high blood pressure and signs of damage to other organ systems, often the liver and kidneys, typically occurring after 20 weeks of gestation.

Preterm Pregnancy: A pregnancy that reaches 20 weeks but delivers before 37 completed weeks of gestation.

Second Trimester: The middle stage of pregnancy, covering weeks 13 to 26.

Shoulder Dystocia: A delivery complication where one or both of the babys shoulders become lodged inside the mothers pelvis during vaginal delivery.

SGA (Small for Gestational Age): A fetus or newborn whose weight is below the 10th percentile for their gestational age.

SROM (Spontaneous Rupture of Membranes): The natural breaking of the amniotic sac, leading to the release of amniotic fluid, commonly called the "water breaking."

Sternum: The breastbone, located in the center of the chest, connects the rib bones.

Sutures/Stitches: Materials surgeons use to hold tissue together after an incision or injury, facilitating healing.

SVE (Sterile Vaginal Exam): A manual examination of the vagina and cervix performed under sterile conditions to assess labor progress.

Third Trimester: The final stage of pregnancy, from week 27 to birth.

TOLAC (Trial of Labor After Cesarean): An attempt to have a vaginal birth after a previous Cesaren

www.ingramcontent.com/pod-product-compliance
Lightning Source LLC
LaVergne TN
LVHW011520200926
848484LV00001B/90